T0202111

In the Aftermath of the Pandemic

In the Aftermath
of the Pandemic

Interpersonal Psychotherapy for Anxiety,
Depression, and PTSD

JOHN C. MARKOWITZ

OXFORD
UNIVERSITY PRESS

OXFORD
UNIVERSITY PRESS

Oxford University Press is a department of the University of Oxford. It furthers
the University's objective of excellence in research, scholarship, and education
by publishing worldwide. Oxford is a registered trade mark of Oxford University
Press in the UK and certain other countries.

Published in the United States of America by Oxford University Press
198 Madison Avenue, New York, NY 10016, United States of America.

© Oxford University Press 2021

All rights reserved. No part of this publication may be reproduced, stored in
a retrieval system, or transmitted, in any form or by any means, without the
prior permission in writing of Oxford University Press, or as expressly permitted
by law, by license, or under terms agreed with the appropriate reproduction
rights organization. Inquiries concerning reproduction outside the scope of the
above should be sent to the Rights Department, Oxford University Press, at the
address above.

You must not circulate this work in any other form
and you must impose this same condition on any acquirer.

Library of Congress Cataloging-in-Publication Data

Names: Markowitz, John C., 1954- author.
Title: In the aftermath of the pandemic : interpersonal psychotherapy for
    anxiety, depression, and PTSD / John C. Markowitz.
Description: New York, NY : Oxford University Press, [2021] | Includes
    bibliographical references and index.
Identifiers: LCCN 2020054638 (print) | LCCN 2020054639 (ebook) |
    ISBN 9780197554500 (paperback) | ISBN 9780197554524 (epub) |
    ISBN 9780197554531
Subjects: LCSH: Interpersonal psychotherapy. | COVID-19
    (Disease)—Psychological aspects. | Disasters—Psychological aspects. |
    Stress management.
Classification: LCC RC489.I55 M347 2021 (print) | LCC RC489.I55 (ebook) |
    DDC 616.2/4140651—dc23
LC record available at https://lccn.loc.gov/2020054638
LC ebook record available at https://lccn.loc.gov/2020054639

DOI: 10.1093/med-psych/9780197554500.001.0001

9 8 7 6 5 4 3 2

Printed by Marquis, Canada

Dedicated to the incomprehensible numbers of the dead, of the still living and suffering, and to those struggling to help them

CONTENTS

Introduction

The Pandemic

In 2020 the world suddenly and seemingly irrevocably changed. The Covid-19 virus, previously unknown, often lethal, and without a treatment, began to devastate populations around the globe. In the absence of a vaccine, societies retreated to ancient patterns of plague control, namely social distancing. This physical isolation protected individuals, kept intensive care units (ICUs) from overflowing, and limited at least the speed of infection—but at a cost.

The anti-Covid lockdown in the United States saved lives, at least in parts of the country that obeyed it. It brought with it, however, a host of problems: loss of sense of health safety, and sometimes loss of health itself; loss of daily routine, loss of social support, loss of income, often loss of job, and sometimes loss of loved ones (see Table I.1). These losses, alone and combined, contributed to the next and, we fear, enduring wave of pathology during the spread and in the wake of the Covid-19 virus. We anticipate, and seem already to be seeing,[1] psychopathology on a grand scale: anxiety, depression, traumatic stress, and substance misuse. Those who haven't died or become physically ill still suffer.

In the midst of this pandemic, our team of psychiatric researchers at Columbia University/New York State Psychiatric Institute (NYSPI) sought to provide remote (virtual, phone and internet video) treatment to patients in need. Remote therapy is itself a major adjustment for therapists used to seeing patients in person.[2] And a major adjustment for patients, too. Moreover, it was unclear whether the treatment lessons we had learned from other traumatic events, such as rape, war, the September 11 attacks, and natural disasters like hurricanes and earthquakes, applied to this catastrophe. Most traumatic events are, thankfully, brief, whereas this pandemic is (as I write in May 2020) already a siege that promises to continue. Prolonged stress is more distressing and becomes more engrained than acute stress.[3] The longer it continues, the worse the effects. And while the Covid-19 "plague" is an impersonal trauma, which is comparatively less distressing than interpersonal trauma,[4,5] its extreme interpersonal consequences compound its damage.

Table I.1. LOSSES DUE TO THE COVID-19 PANDEMIC ENGENDER PSYCHIATRIC
SYMPTOMS

Loss	Threat	Consequences
Loss of security	Potentially lethal viral infection Frontline medical and other personnel witness trauma	Fear of or actual illness → anxiety, pain, PTSD, depression, anxiety
Loss of income	Anxiety about rent, food, finances	Anxiety, depression
Loss of employment	Damage to career, income	Anxiety, depression
Loss of loved ones	Complicated mourning	Traumatic loss; disrupted mourning rituals → anxiety, depression, PTSD
Loss of routine	Home lockdown	Disrupted social rhythms, activities, pleasures → anxiety, depression
Loss of social support	Physical distancing can mean social isolation	Social isolation → anxiety, depression

A further layer of interpersonal malignity magnifies the effects of corona-virus. From the start of the pandemic, Americans have seen other countries, led by unifying, compassionate leaders, take orchestrated, scientifically driven steps to combat the spread of infection, with often beneficial results. In contrast, the U.S. federal government has been divisive, attacking, openly racist at a moment when racial and ethnic minorities are hardest hit, and strikingly anti-scientific. The President of the United States has recommended unproven and dangerous remedies such as injecting bleach (!) and turned wearing a mask into a polit-ical statement rather than a public health measure. The federal and many state governments have failed on many levels, for many people, their leaders pointedly ignoring and discounting a rising plague in defiance of basic medical tenets. Spike Lee made the point in his 2006 film *When the Levees Broke* that although Hurricane Katrina was an impersonal trauma, the failed, racist governmental response to the disaster gave it added interpersonal insult.

Amidst the pandemic, in the anticipation of a polarized national election, there has been a sudden explosion of national awareness and protest about structural racism following airings of videotaped evidence of the killings of George Floyd on May 25, 2020, and other African American men and women, by white policemen. The Black Lives Matter movement is a healthy, belated response to centuries of in-equality and mistreatment, and its invigoration seems a healthy channeling of the frustrations of months of lockdown into an idealistic cause. Dealing with struc-tural racism is an important cause, albeit not the focus of this book. Nonetheless, all this change adds to the turmoil in the environment individuals face.

Moreover, this is only the first wave of virus, and first aftershock of psychiatric symptoms. If there are future waves, as it appears there may well be, they will likely compound the psychiatric sequelae. What effect will this pandemic have not only on the adults who lose their jobs, but also on their children who are evicted from their schools and separated from their friends for months on end? Even after a vaccine arrives, the psychiatric consequences of this global disaster will likely be long-lasting.

This book describes the application of interpersonal psychotherapy (IPT) to treating the psychiatric consequences of Covid-19, and more generally to any terrible social disaster. IPT is one of many psychotherapies, and it is surely not the only route to treating post-Covid psychological symptoms, but many therapists and patients may find it a particularly useful approach.[6] I will explain why in a moment.

Most books on IPT have followed a research data stream. Almost every IPT adaptation for a particular psychiatric disorder has been empirically tested and shown to work before it has been disseminated. We know that IPT benefits people with major depressive disorder (MDD),[7,8] bipolar disorder (adapted as interpersonal social rhythms therapy [IPSRT]),[9] eating disorders,[7] and posttraumatic stress disorder (PTSD).[3,10,11] What we don't entirely know is how much it helps people who develop distress, depression, or PTSD in the wake of a prolonged disaster such as the Covid pandemic. We hope that the National Institute of Mental Health, which has in recent years funded neuroscience at the expense of clinical research,[12] will recognize the need for immediate clinical trials as a result of the mental health fallout of the pandemic. Nonetheless, as we await research evidence, IPT appears to be a good candidate for the psychiatric consequences of disaster. All of the treatment cases described in this book, while disguised to protect patient confidentiality, are actual presentations from the pandemic.

Why should IPT work in the setting of disaster? First, IPT has been shown to alleviate MDD and PTSD, two of the most common sequelae of traumatic life events, and to lower anxiety. Second, IPT is a life event–based therapy, using life circumstances to contextualize psychiatric crises, explain strong emotional reactions, and use understanding of those emotions to negotiate interpersonal and other life difficulties.[7] The worse the life circumstances, the more understandable strong feelings become. A pandemic is surely a life event, and it brings other distressing events—unemployment, financial need, strained interpersonal relationships, etc.—in its trail. Third, IPT focuses on mobilizing interpersonal support and on repairing attachment.[13,14] This makes it an appropriate intervention for a time of interpersonal isolation, when physical separation threatens to deprive individuals of needed social support.[6] Social support is a key protection against anxiety, depression, PTSD, and psychic and medical vulnerability more generally.[5] Fourth, the loss of daily structure contributes to people's disorientation and discomfort during the crisis. Adding components of social rhythms therapy (from interpersonal social rhythms therapy[15]) can help to restore the lost structure of pre-Covid daily life.

People often don't like to have strong feelings, particularly negative feelings. Because of that discomfort, they often try to minimize their feelings through intellectualization, distraction, or suppression. The Covid pandemic inevitably evokes powerful feelings, and particularly "negative" affects such as anxiety, anger, and sadness. Some of these feelings are appropriate to the situation, others excessive. A precept of IPT is that feelings are important and informative: it is better to know how you feel, and why, in order to respond to life's situations. It's important to recognize that painful affects can be normal: they reflect a painful environment.[3] When feelings go unrecognized and detached from context, they can become a confusing additional internal pressure for an individual to struggle with.

All of these features suggest IPT as a helpful counterweight to the stresses of the pandemic.[6] We are using IPT at Columbia/New York Psychiatric Institute as well as in private practice to assess its benefits, and thus far it seems quite helpful. I hope that the reader, who is likely a psychotherapist treating patients with various emotional and psychiatric responses to these painful events, will agree.

John C. Markowitz, MD
May 2020

An update at the completion of the text: three months later, Covid-19 has not begun to disappear. While New York is no longer the American epicenter of the virus, more than three million Americans have already been infected, more than 130,000 have died, and the daily number of new infections is rising. We are in for a longer siege than anticipated, with growing psychiatric consequences.

July 2020

1

In the Aftermath of Upheaval

Our environment shapes us. Here in the United States, protected by two broad oceans, we had long been spared threats of invasion. Geography may have fostered a sense of security that partially explains the long-standing American ethos of confidence.[16] Things have become shakier of late, however, since the September 11, 2001 attacks and now the invasion of an invisible, potentially lethal killer. As the world becomes more threatening, we feel more threatened.

THE DISASTER

Beginning in March 2020, the country and the world turned upside down. Americans began dying in incomprehensibly large numbers—more than 100,000 before the end of May. Many who didn't die became seriously and chronically ill. The symptoms of Covid-19 took a while to fully appreciate, but it quickly became clear that acute respiratory distress often required ventilator support, and hospital ICUs became overloaded. With closed borders disrupting supply lines, a shortage arose of personal protective equipment (PPE) such as face masks and gloves, as well as access to viral testing. In the finest, most sophisticated hospitals in the world's richest nation, doctors, nurses, and other staff were forced to reuse PPE, often inadvertently infecting patients and themselves. Bodies have piled up in refrigerated trucks as morgues have overflowed. The initial public reaction was, understandably, fear (albeit, in some quarters, denial).

Frontline medical workers are facing particular risk of infection. Poorer, minority communities, with denser housing and poorer access to treatment and whose work often put them at risk for contagion, are suffering disproportionate illness and death. So are the elderly, particularly debilitated individuals clustered in nursing homes, and inpatients in psychiatric hospitals.

While medical professionals around the country and the world have pulled together impressively to provide patients supportive treatment of Covid-19 symptoms and to study potential treatments and vaccines, the infection has no immediate cure. Protecting lives hence requires isolation, quarantine, and social distancing. When the virus struck, businesses, restaurants, and entertainment closed. The economy ground to a near halt. Unemployment figures in the United States reached almost forty million (40,000,000) in a matter of weeks, with unemployment rates rising from 3.5% to almost 15%. People worried about how to pay the rent and to obtain food to eat. Food banks were overwhelmed by miles-long lines of cars. The federal government's response to this catastrophic situation was and (months later!) remains disorganized, inadequate, and often counterproductive, leaving each state to fend for itself. It has been shocking and surreal to see New York City shift abruptly from bustling megalopolis to sci-fi ghost town (Figure 1.1).

Many frontline individuals caring for patients are risking their own lives and witnessing horrible events and deaths, the "Criterion A" of the fifth edition of the *Diagnostic and Statistical Manual of Mental Disorders* (DSM-5) traumas that qualify for the diagnosis of PTSD.[17] Compounding this has often been a sense of moral injury that lack of supplies and of governmental support is sabotaging their work and putting their patients' and their own lives at unnecessary risk.[18]

Even the many Americans who have had asymptomatic infection or avoided the virus suffer. There has been a torrent of upsetting news, evoking upsetting feelings. Each of the medical and social stressors listed in Table I.1 would have sufficed to produce high levels of anxiety in the general population and, as time has dragged on in months of isolation, to breed frustration and depression and eventually boredom from the monotony. The pent-up frustration may have contributed to subsequent crowd violence. Attempts at the "reopening" of limited

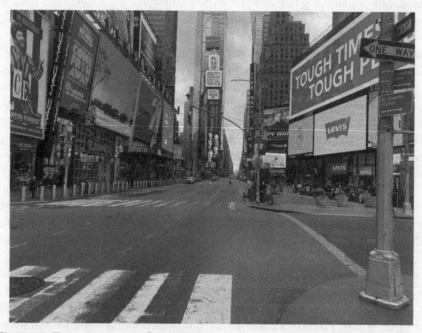

Figure 1.1 Times Square, March 31, 2020.
Photo by the author.

social life and business, a seemingly encouraging development, have brought new fears and realities of infectious spread. Two other central factors have extended from and compounded the anomaly of the situation: the social and economic lockdown required by social distancing disrupted social rhythms and social support.

Disruption of Social Rhythms

Part of what makes normal life normal is a familiar daily routine. Most people fare best waking up at the same hour every morning, sitting down to coffee and break-fast; then commuting to work, interacting with colleagues, and following work protocols until the time comes to return home. Then preparing dinner, eating, and spending time with one's family, perhaps watching television or reading before heading for bed—again, often at a set hour. The temporal and behavioral landmarks of such a day, termed *social zeitgebers*, or "time givers," help give us our social role and orient us to the environment.[19] Such social rhythms provide a comfortable psychic structure to the day as well as conditioning a regular, healthy somatic sleep cycle.

We all rely on these patterns. Individuals with bipolar disorders are particularly sensitive to such daily stimuli, which is why interpersonal social rhythms treatment (IPSRT)[9,15] was developed for their treatment. Disrupting familiar life patterns is disorienting and anxiety-provoking, particularly when the pattern shifts very suddenly for the whole population. Who am I if I'm not going to my job? How do I define my day and week if I'm stuck at home all the time? During the lockdown, not just personal patterns but also larger social patterns ceased. Public spaces and activities closed. There were no longer sports scores to check. Outside entertainment and restaurants shut down. Stores closed or had limited access, leading to runs on toilet paper and other supplies because things we took for granted could no longer be so.

While some individuals who could still work from home initially felt pleased not to have to commute, for many this pleasure quickly waned. Days lost their structure. There was no longer a boundary between work and home life, making it hard to unwind from stressful work. Parents whose children's schools had closed struggled to work (if they still had work), teach, and simultaneously provide child care in the course of the day. College students were forced to return home, feeling cheated of their collegiate experience, distanced from their classmates, and unhappily stuck with their families at a moment of expected independence. With the breakdown in routine, many people began to feel disoriented and uncomfortable: "surreal" was an adjective frequently used. Life was no longer normal, and the abnormality was unnerving. With limited options for activity, people grew increasingly frustrated and bored.

These disruptions in schedule frequently interfered with and disrupted sleep schedules, leaving people tired, more irritable, and more anxious. All this disruption is fertile soil for distress and psychopathology.

Social Distancing and Social Support

The requirement to "shelter in place" meant having to stay home. This physical isolation of quarantine tended to cut people off from friends, family, and work colleagues, from confidants and acquaintances. Thus physical isolation risked loss of social support. As people are social animals, this isolation was palpable. Zoom parties and phone conversations compensated a bit, the "seven o'clock cheer" that rang through cities every evening to salute healthcare workers provided a bit of communal solidarity, but mostly people felt cut off.[20] Even when meeting in person, behind masks and gloves, six foot social distancing meant the absence of physical contact; people missed hugs and kisses.

Social support is a crucial factor in mental and even physical health.[5,21,22] Social isolation has been linked to physical decline and premature death.[23] Social support means that you do not feel alone, that if you have problems and strong feelings you can share them with others, rather than keeping them in as painful secrets. Feeling anxious or depressed by various losses or other aspects of the pandemic, people were (and remain, at this writing) threatened with loss of part of the security system that stabilized their lives. Everyone has suffered, but people with already limited social support, already at higher risk for psychiatric symptoms, have suffered more.

A further problem has arisen. In the absence of the usual patterns of life, many people have turned, understandably, to virtual life. The internet provides endless diversion, news, fake news, and social media contacts to those who seek them. Keeping track of some news seems only healthy, to know what is going on so as to be able to respond. Yet it has become clear that too much social media use is a risk factor for psychiatric symptoms, ranging from anxiety to depression to suicide risk.[24-31]

THE SECOND WAVE: PSYCHOPATHOLOGY IN THE WAKE OF THE PANDEMIC

Thus, overnight, normal life became extremely abnormal. It remains so months later. Essentially everyone has felt stresses and suffered losses, generating anxiety, sadness, anger, and other feelings. Some of that has been warranted: anxiety, based on fear of infection, fear of an uncertain future. Sadness, reflecting loss. Anger at the frustrations of a circumscribed life, at missed opportunities, and at others in a crowded household living one on top of another. Although most people are resilient in adjusting to stressors, finding some way to roll with the punches, a substantial subset will suffer symptoms (Figure 1.2). The greater the concatenation of stressors, and the longer they persist, the greater the likelihood and severity of psychiatric symptoms.

Our PTSD team at Columbia University/NYSPI, led by my colleague Yuval Neria, PhD, remembered the psychiatric aftereffects of the September 11, 2001

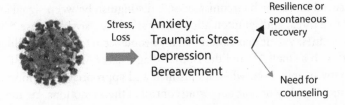

Most people will be resilient.

Figure 1.2 Psychological fallout of the Covid-19 pandemic.

World Trade Center attack and became immediately concerned that the viral pandemic would trigger a large and long-lasting second wave of psychopathology.[32] In retrospect, 9/11 was a brief if horrific trauma, yet its scars persist to this day. While most people adjusted to it, individuals vulnerable to trauma (based on prior trauma, genetics, or psychiatric history) or severe exposure to the trauma (e.g., proximity to the World Trade Center, knowing someone who died in the towers) developed PTSD, major depression, substance misuse, or some combination of these.[33] In the current pandemic, we felt there were just too many stressors, too many losses, affecting the entire populace for too long. Even as the first viral wave seemed to begin to recede, a new wave of psychiatric disorders was likely to follow.

Disorders could result from stressors or possibly even from central nervous system effects of Covid-19 infection itself.[34] Frontline clinicians trying to provide care face high risk. An upsetting headline in New York City on April 27, 2020 was the suicide of Dr. Lorna Breen, the forty-nine-year-old medical director of the emergency department at New York–Presbyterian Allen Hospital in Upper Manhattan, an epicenter within the epicenter of the viral assault.[35] Dr. Breen had contracted Covid-19, gone home to recuperate for some ten days, and then perhaps rushed back to her emergency room (ER) service too soon. She again witnessed scores of unpreventable deaths in an overwhelmed system. The hospital again sent her home, after which she killed herself.

HOW SHOULD YOU FEEL?

Context matters: life events have emotional consequences. In a moment of great tumult, feelings grow tumultuous too. Anxiety is a normal response to threat, and the pandemic is a threat. Sadness is a normal response to loss, and people are suffering losses. Anger is a normal response to frustration, and these are frustrating times of curtailed lives. As psychotherapists surely know, people often have difficulty gauging whether their feelings are appropriate, whether they can trust their own feelings. Most of us do not like strong affects, and particularly negative affects. Under such novel and unpleasant circumstances, it is small wonder that people would struggle to tolerate their emotional responses.

It is crucial under such circumstances to distinguish between signal anxiety as the alert to a threat and symptomatic anxiety as an excessive response.[36] The same holds for sadness versus depression—many people seem to confuse colloquial "depression" with a small "d" and the DSM-5 diagnosis of Major Depression. Anger scares many people, even when it's justified and appropriate, still more if it gets out of hand. People worry about losing control of their emotions. Yet the question under these circumstances is not whether one should feel anxious, angry, or sad but how strongly it's helpful to feel such things and how to handle those feelings.

Thus, at Columbia/NYSPI we expected a range of psychological reactions to the Covid-19 pandemic, depending upon individual experiences, histories, and vulnerabilities (Figure 1.2). Everyone was stressed, and everyone would surely be anxious at first and increasingly frustrated and demoralized as the siege dragged on. We expected that most people would be resilient, as most people—remarkably—bounce back even in the face of great stress.[37,38] Resilience, "the process of adapting well in the face of adversity, trauma, tragedy, threats or significant sources of stress,"[39] is a complex, important phenomenon described at length in Chapter 9 of this book. Humans are adaptable creatures, and we tend to roll with life's circumstances. On the other hand, we expected the usual response to severe stress in vulnerable individuals. People would respond as they often did under stress: people with eating disorders might have heightened eating problems; those with trichotillomania might pull out more hair. The big quartet of syndromes were likely to be anxiety, depression, PTSD, and substance use disorders, some of them recurrences but others arising *de novo* based on exposure to recent circumstances. Our program is not set up to treat substance disorders, but we certainly have seen heightened PTSD, depression, and anxiety disorders. So has my private practice, with some long absent patients returning with recurrent symptoms, and others arriving with new ones. Unfortunately, even if life returns to something approaching "normal," we can expect to keep seeing these psychiatric aftershocks for some time to come.

2

How the Pandemic Has Transformed Psychotherapy

Remote Treatment

While the pandemic has put millions of Americans out of work, therapists are finding plenty to do. People need psychological support and treatment. The problem has been that social distancing directly affects the practice of psychotherapy, it being no longer safe to have patient and therapist share an enclosed space for the prolonged interval of a treatment session. As a result, everything has gone remote: tele-psychiatry has taken over.* The delivery of IPT, as described in this book, will for the foreseeable future mean remote, tele-IPT.

Tele-psychiatry has been around in one form or another for decades.[40] The term "tele-psychiatry" is broad and vague, encompassing telephone therapy, smartphone or computer videotherapy, as well as computer-driven programs and internet apps. Until now, tele-psychiatry had mainly been used to help hard-to-reach populations who lacked access to in-person treatment: rural HIV-positive patients,[41] for example, rural military veterans far from Veteran Affairs (VA) hospitals, and nursing home patients. Whereas in-person effective psychotherapies have been extensively studied, with more than a thousand studies of MDD alone,[42] the corresponding database for tele-psychiatry of any kind, for any disorder, is quite limited.[2]

Even the existing research has limitations. Many published studies were underpowered to show differences, or influenced by researcher enthusiasm for tele-therapy, leading to potentially biased outcomes. Moreover, because many researchers and their institutional review boards felt understandable discomfort

---

* Note: This chapter is based upon Markowitz JC, Milrod B, Heckman TG, Bergman M, Amsalem D, Zalman H, Ballas T, Neria Y: On remote: psychotherapy at a distance *Am J Psychiatry* 2020;177 Epub ahead of print 25 Sep 2020. https://doi.org/10.1176/appi.ajp.2020.20050557. Adapted with permission from the American Journal of Psychiatry (Copyright © 2020). American Psychiatric Association. All Rights Reserved.

about treating high risk psychiatric patients at a distance, many research trials excluded highly symptomatic patients, yielding more mildly ill treatment samples. Yet because milder symptoms tend to respond to almost any benign treatment, including placebo,[43] the common report that tele-therapy has comparable outcomes to in-person therapy should be skeptically received. The extant evidence appears stronger for the benefits of telephone therapy than for videotherapy, for which trials have been scarce. In any event, such research as exists is an inadequate foundation to support the sudden massive use of tele-therapy, and particularly videotherapy, as standard treatment.[2]

Yet overnight, tele-therapy became standard treatment nonetheless. This has required considerable adjustment for therapists. Our Columbia/NYSPI group, which had previously used telephone psychotherapy and tele-videotherapy in selected circumstances for patients with transportation difficulties, compared among ourselves our current experiences and agreed that remote therapy presents numerous issues. These relate to setting, transmission, physical discomfort, and emotional distancing (Table 2.1).

The great strength of remote therapy is that it expands access: the great majority of Americans have access to a telephone or computer.[44,45] Nonetheless, recent reports suggest that many at-risk populations, including the poor and the elderly, often lack high-speed internet access.[46-48] At least one formerly homeless patient we had been treating in person declined to continue therapy even by phone because sessions would have cost him precious billed minutes on his phone plan. Several other patients reported lacking any private space to speak away from difficult family members in cramped, overstuffed apartments. Remote therapy has the great benefit of maintaining a therapeutic connection and allowing treatment

Table 2.1 REMOTE THERAPY DIFFICULTIES AND POTENTIAL REMEDIES

Difficulty	Remedy
Setting Teletherapy Your home background	Acknowledge difference from in-person Arrange to minimize distraction, disclosure
Transmission difficulties	Bear with interruptions
Physical Intrusions	"Try to find a private place where you are unlikely to be overheard or interrupted . . ." Observe patient's environment
Electronic intrusions Email beeps Your own face "Talking heads"	Turn off email (and ask patient to) Minimize or hide self-view Sit at in-person session distance, away from keyboard
Physical discomfort	Relax, stretch between sessions Use a comfortable, ergonomic chair
Emotional distancing	Minimize outside distractions Focus on reading patient

to continue at a time of great need. In reaching patients, however, remote therapy requires important adjustments for therapists, on several levels. As therapists and supervisors, we sense great differences treating patients with psychotherapy by webcam or telephone rather than in person.

SETTING

Many clinics that have practiced telepsychiatry, including ours,[49-51] had required at least one initial in-person visit to evaluate the patient and develop a therapeutic alliance before continuing treatment remotely. That is no longer practical or safe: now treatment is distanced from the start. This may subtly alter the therapeutic relationship. Nor can one offer a tearful patient a tissue. Patients who began therapy in-person and had anticipated it would continue can find the adjustment to remote therapy "weird" (as several said) and discomfiting, although they soon seem to settle in. Therapists may, too.

Maintaining a consistent intimate focus is more difficult. The patient is no longer in the room but on a screen (or a phone). Instead of two human beings fully engaging in a common space, one meets an image of a patient on a computer screen (or a disembodied voice) surrounded by too many distracting stimuli. Although studies indicate good therapeutic alliance and psychotherapeutic common factors can be established in remote therapies,[52-54] they may reflect selective, enthusiastic therapist and patient samples.

Distractions abound. The usual instruction to patients is to find a private, quiet space where the patient is unlikely to be overheard or interrupted, but that is not always possible, particularly for less privileged patients under lockdown. People and pets walk in. Outside noises distract. Even if they do not, the screens themselves teem with diversions. Because the computer volume is on (sometimes set very loud) to allow therapist–patient interchange, the frequent ping of arriving email occurs at both venues. We have seen patients scanning the screen as if reading an email, rather than making eye contact. Eye contact itself is tricky: if the patient is addressing the computer camera lens, making virtual eye contact, he or she may not be looking at your image; and vice versa. Thus the patient's gaze may be misleading. Your own image on your screen is an anomalous presence: you or your patient may be looking at oneself rather than each other.

Instead of sitting close to the camera, viewing each other as talking heads, you can sit back, and ask the patient to sit back, providing more of a full-length view, a simulacrum of the office experience. This also distances yourselves from the keyboard to avoid the temptation of email. Some video programs have a "hide self-view" option or can enlarge the patient view relative to self-view, allowing a purer focus on the patient. These maneuvers may reduce unhelpful sensory stimuli. On the other hand, too much distance from the microphone can hurt sound quality, and headphones can be obtrusive. The issues video treatment raises suggest that telephone therapy might present fewer distractions, albeit at the therapeutic cost of nonverbal cues, particularly for patients unable to easily express their feelings in words.

Remote therapy grants the therapist revealing glimpses of a patient's home and life. This may include meeting pets, babies, and other family members, and seeing elements in the surroundings that the patient might not think to mention. One patient appeared in her childhood bedroom, where a devout religious icon hung on the wall. She had mentioned having been raised in a "kind of religious, Catholic" home, but the camera brought her mother's consuming devout piety, and graphic reminders of the strictures this imposes on the patient's life, into sharp relief. Other patients could only find private space in a bathroom, on the stairs of her building, or outside in a park.

Most patients seem not to mind allowing their therapists into their homes, although those preoccupied with their outward appearance, hoarders ashamed of their household interiors, and some mistrustful patients with social anxiety disorder or PTSD have requested telephone rather than video sessions. Anecdotal conversations with colleagues suggest that more than half of their patients prefer standard telephones to videophones for remote therapy purposes. One patient personalized her screen background to surround herself with a family portrait. A therapist noted that some patients have been conditioned to feel a work ethic in front of their computer screen, and seem more relaxed on the telephone. Just as good therapists offer patients informed consent and a choice of treatment modality, remote therapists might offer patients a choice of treatment medium: i.e., telephone or video.

For their part, some therapists feel odd about treating patients from their own personal spaces (e.g., a bedroom), to which a crowded house may confine them. It may be important to pre-check the camera frame so as to avoid unwanted, inadvertent self-disclosure of personal home details. Whereas many therapists do not miss commuting to work, they note in retrospect that it provided time to decompress and think through the progress of treatments prior to rejoining private or family life. That transitional buffer may no longer exist when one works from home. It may help to allot time to reflect before and after treatment sessions to ease the shift to domestic life. During the Covid-19 crisis, however, many people lack extra time as details of domestic life have become more burdensome.[55]

PHYSICAL DISCOMFORT

Everyone in our group has found remote psychotherapy more physically and psychically exhausting than the in-person variety. Many therapists on our academic listservs have volunteered the same response. There are several apparent reasons. It is harder to stay focused on and more difficult to read the patient's cues across the medium. Sitting before a screen constricts physical movement, including the subconscious mirroring movements in which patients and therapists sharing a space engage. Therapists feel rigidly locked before the camera, tensing different muscles. It can feel like, and have the physical consequences, of a long haul airline flight. We encourage therapists to use comfortable, ergonomic desk chairs and to stretch their legs and bodies and walk around their house between sessions to counter this.

TRANSMISSION

Technical difficulties can impede communication or interrupt treatment sessions: difficulty connecting, frozen screens, unstable internet warnings, garbled or delayed audio, poor lighting, dropped calls. Videotherapy has turned out to have confidentiality risks, although it can be HIPAA-secured.[56] Time spent countering these inefficiencies means less time for engagement in therapy.

EMOTIONAL DISTANCING

Perhaps the greatest challenge in remote therapy is a loss of affective nuance on the telephone or screen. This factor that seems to bother therapists more than patients (albeit we have not solicited patient reactions). The affective diminution makes the experience less emotionally vibrant, particularly for patients with the psychological tendency to dissociate. Media separation makes it hard to gauge nonverbal behavioral subtleties,[57] such as when a patient with PTSD may be dissociating. A pause on the phone can mean (too) many things. Although research has found tele-exposure therapy benefits patients,[58,59] it seems easier for patients to avoid exposure at geographic and interpersonal distance. In affect-focused psychotherapies, distance impedes emotional engagement with the therapist in the moment, which is key to the process of change. We have arrived at no solution to this problem except to minimize distractions and to work hard to focus on understanding the patient's emotional state.

Patients who participate in tele-therapy in the familiar "safety" of their home, particularly those with anxiety, panic, and agoraphobia, may underreport symptoms likely to be present (or activated) when presenting in clinical venues. Thus physical remoteness appears to aggravate these patients' avoidance of uncomfortable affects and experiences.

THE PANDEMIC

It would deny reality to pretend that current tele-therapy is therapy as usual. The Covid-19 pandemic is a world crisis, and it tends to aggravate underlying anxiety in at least three ways: (1) by evoking appropriate fears of contagion, which may rapidly merge into panic attacks (anxiety as signal versus symptom)[36]; (2) by disrupting the comfortable structure and rhythm of the patient's (and therapist's) work and life schedule, often including where and with whom they are living, and sources of income and relaxation; and (3) through social distancing, which stretches attachment bonds and risks loss of social support.[6] As the pandemic has persisted, initial panic in the general population seems to be giving way to frustration, despondency, and depression for many, with concern that suicide risk may be increasing.[60] As in previous pandemics[61] and disasters,[62] highly exposed groups such as medical teams, first responders, and the bereaved may well present with lingering PTSD and complicated grief.

Therapists should acknowledge the crisis, and perhaps that tele-therapy is a limited substitute for more direct contact. They can attempt to maintain the helpful structure of therapy by maintaining regular sessions and treatment approach. They can encourage patients to maximize their existing relationships by remote means to preserve protective social support.[6]

The pandemic not only evokes new symptoms but functions as a Rorschach test, magnifying aspects of patients' ongoing inner struggles. People respond to crisis in varying, idiosyncratic ways. Patients with obsessive compulsive disorder have joked that the world has finally caught up to them on handwashing. Embarrassing behavioral differences between severely agoraphobic and social phobic patients and "normal people" have temporarily shrunk. Some depressed patients have become more depressed, whereas others say the crisis has led them to downgrade their previous concerns: that Covid-19 has been de-catastrophizing, as it were. A severely symptomatic veteran with PTSD who had been in productive, exploratory, trauma-focused psychodynamic psychotherapy,[63] became distanced, repeatedly telling his therapist that all symptoms were "just the same," that "nothing's new really" once his treatment switched to videotherapy. He evidently said this in response to an unspoken or unconscious urge to protect her from his rage-filled fantasies and recurrent dreams after having learned early in the pandemic that she required isolation (earlier than other VA employees required it) because of an immune-compromising illness. This patient began to improve, and use therapy more productively, only after the therapist pointed out this seeming attempt to protect her. The therapist had uncharacteristically avoided making this observation for several stymied weeks because of her own concerns about being less available to the patient remotely than she would have been in person.

CONCLUSIONS

Several modalities of tele-therapy can preserve the crucially important link of psychotherapy in a highly anxiety- and depression-provoking, socially burdened time of quarantine, social distancing, and deep emotional need and despair. Tele-therapy has some empirical backing, but the outcome literature is very limited relative to that of in-person treatment and has unclear generalizability to its broad current use among a wide range of patients with various serious psychiatric problems. Tele-psychotherapy offers access and convenience during a time of unprecedented crisis, at the cost of important elements of in-person treatment. At least in the United States, Covid-19 has changed the long-standing requirement that therapists see patients in person. This may well change the face of psychotherapy and enhance the ongoing use of tele-therapy, whether or not it is an optimal approach. Our experience to date suggests that in-person psychotherapy, now necessarily in limbo, has many advantages over remote treatment and should eventually return.

It is unclear whether videotherapy, despite its sudden wide uptake, is necessarily clinically preferable to telephone therapy. The limited empirical research does not demonstrate the superiority of video treatment. Vision, as the dominant human sense, may have prejudiced insurance reimbursement requirements for visual patient tele-contact (when insurance has paid for videotherapy at all[64]). Video has obvious advantages over audio for group therapy, but it may provide more distractions than a simple phone call for some or many patients in individual therapy. Such preference, which can affect treatment outcome,[65,66] deserves study. Telephone may also provide broader access to economically disadvantaged patients. Perhaps insurance should reimburse both media: tele-therapy research sparked by Covid-19 could reveal that what has always been an arbitrary insurance requirement is in fact an unnecessary one.

Covid-19 will eventually be contained and the world will resume some new form of normalcy. Nonetheless, coronavirus may continue to have ongoing effects on social closeness and on how (remotely) psychotherapy is practiced. The wave of viral contagion may pass, only to be followed by a wave of psychopathology. Inasmuch as previous, far more contained disasters have raised the incidence of anxiety, mood, PTSD, and substance use, Covid-19 likely will as well.

Another historical complication of tele-therapy has been that each of the fifty United States required therapist licensure in the patient's state of residence. This legal requirement greatly impeded a central strength of remote therapy, namely its broad and relatively inexpensive geographic reach. In response to the pandemic, the federal government in March 2020 relaxed this obligation, allowing therapists to treat patients across state lines.[67] Hopefully this freedom to cross boundaries will continue after the pandemic passes.

3

Interpersonal Psychotherapy

Life Event–Based Therapy

Interpersonal psychotherapy is an evidence-based, time-limited, diagnosis-targeted, affect-focused, patient- and therapist-friendly psychotherapy. IPT helps patients to understand their feelings as useful guides to interpersonal situations and to use them to resolve a current crisis related to their underlying disorder. People don't like life difficulties and often don't like the strong feelings that arise from them. Nor do they always understand their interplay. In the time-limited space of a dozen weeks or so, IPT helps patients to tolerate and understand their feelings, use them to resolve a seemingly overwhelming life crisis, mobilize protective social support, and thus gain mastery over both internal emotion and external reality. Patients set their own pace, without formal homework, but are pushed to action by the pressure of the time limit. Patients tend to like IPT, making dropout low compared to exposure-based treatments.

The pandemic, like any disaster, surely provides life events to work on. Whereas cognitive behavioral therapy (CBT) benefits from the disparity between a relatively benign life situation and catastrophic thinking, IPT works best in the setting of actual trouble. In an (in-person) randomized controlled study comparing IPT and CBT as for depressed patients with human immunodeficiency virus (HIV) infection at the height of the AIDS epidemic, we found advantages for IPT over CBT.[68] When life is in fact catastrophic, it provides a powerful explanatory rationale for strong feelings and for the appearance of symptoms. So in a sense, IPT therapists like to discover bad events in a patient's history.

This brief handbook cannot describe IPT as comprehensively as in other publications detailing its theory[69,70] and empirical basis,[69] techniques and adaptations,[7] or manuals targeting specific diagnoses.[e.g.,3] Suffice it to say that

(1) IPT was developed based on what was known in the 1970s about the relationship between major depression and interpersonal life events;
(2) IPT has been tested each diagnostic step of the way, disorder by disorder, to determine whom it benefits and whom it may not;

(3) a large body of empirical evidence supports IPT as a time-limited treatment for mood disorders,[8,71] eating disorders,[71] and to a lesser degree for anxiety disorders[72] and PTSD.[10,11] It is listed in treatment guidelines for these syndromes. IPT has not shown clear benefit for substance use disorders, nor for anorexia nervosa (a single negative trial). Like other psychotherapies, it has shown limited benefit as a monotherapy for dysthymic disorder, but may provide important social skills as part of combined therapy with antidepressant medication.[73]

(4) IPT not only relieves symptoms but has been shown to enhance interpersonal skills, in contrast to pharmacotherapy, which relieves depressive symptoms without adding skills.[69,74]

What follows is a practical, hands-on approach to IPT for clinicians treating patients affected by Covid-19 or other disasters.

IPT as an acute treatment has three phases: a beginning, middle, and end.[7] The first phase sets the stage for the therapy to follow, defining the patient's psychiatric diagnosis in the setting of his or her life context. The middle phase entails work on resolving a focal interpersonal life crisis, and the final phase integrates and concludes the brief treatment. For patients who need it, a separately contracted continuation or maintenance IPT can follow acute treatment.[75,76]

THE BASIC PARADIGM: THE CONNECTION BETWEEN LIFE EVENTS AND EMOTIONS

IPT is based on a couple of self-evident axioms. The first is that *emotions and symptoms do not arise in a vacuum, but in an interpersonal context.* Good events evoke positive affects (e.g., happiness, excitement); negative events evoke negative affects (sadness, anxiety, anger). Many people have difficulty tolerating negative affects and try to avoid or suppress them, which may backfire. Some individuals are vulnerable to depression, anxiety, PTSD, or other symptoms or disorders based on genetic risk and early childhood environment. For example, growing up with secure attachment provides protection from symptoms based on a stronger social network and greater confidence in using it to seek social support. Individuals with insecure attachment face symptomatic risk.[5,13]

When life is upsetting enough, and when individuals have a particular vulnerability, their emotional response to the upsetting circumstances may go beyond upsetting feelings and spill over into symptoms and disorders. The original IPT paradigm for major depression notes that upsetting events—the death of a significant other (complicated bereavement), a struggle with a significant other (role dispute), or a major life change (role transition)—may trigger depressive symptoms (see Box 3.1), which then impair social and occupational functioning and lead to further negative events. An individual who is not sleeping, struggles to get out of bed, and is concentrating poorly tends to withdraw socially, arrive

Box 3.1

DSM-5 Major Depressive Disorder (ICD code F32.x)

A. Five (or more) of the following symptoms have been present during the same 2-week period and represent a change from previous functioning; at least one of the symptoms is either (1) depressed mod or (2) loss of interest or pleasure.

Note: Do not include symptoms that are clearly attributable to another medical condition.

1. **Depressed mood** most of the day, nearly every day, as indicated by either subjective report (e.g., feels sad, empty, hopeless) or observation made by others (e.g., appears tearful).
2. **Markedly diminished interest or pleasure** in all, or almost all, activities most of the day, nearly every day (as indicated by either subjective account or observation).
3. **Significant weight loss** when not dieting **or weight gain** (e.g., a change of >5% body in a month), or **decrease or increase in appetite** nearly every day.
4. **Insomnia or hypersomnia** nearly every day.
5. **Psychomotor agitation or retardation** nearly every day (observable by others, not merely subjective feelings of restlessness or being slowed down).
6. **Fatigue** or **loss of energy** nearly every day.
7. **Feelings of worthlessness** or **excessive or inappropriate guilt** (which may be delusional) nearly every day (not merely self-reproach or guilt about being sick).
8. **Diminished ability to think or concentrate**, or **indecisiveness**, nearly every day (either by subjective account or as observed by others).
9. **Recurrent thoughts of death** (not just fear of dying), **recurrent suicidal ideation** without a specific plan, or **a suicide attempt** or **specific plan** for committing suicide

Symptoms must cause clinically significant distress or impair function, are not better explained by substance use or another syndrome, and there is no history of a manic or hypomanic episode.

American Psychiatric Association, 2013, pp.160–161; emphasis added.[17] Reprinted with permission from the *Diagnostic and Statistical Manual of Mental Disorders*, Fifth Edition, (Copyright © 2013). American Psychiatric Association. All Rights Reserved.

places late, and work erratically. The negative functioning worsens mood, and vice versa, in a vicious downward cycle (Figure 3.1).

IPT adapted to treat anxiety or PTSD is simply a variation on this theme: those symptoms also arise in the context of distressing life events and impair functioning, and vice versa. Indeed, a traumatic life event is a requirement to qualify for the diagnosis of PTSD. The same focal problem areas (grief, role dispute, and role transition) that apply to depression also seem to suit these symptom patterns, albeit perhaps with differing frequency.[3,72]

Mood and Events Interact

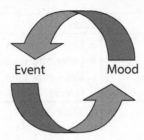

Figure 3.1 Mood and life events interact.

The second principle of IPT is the *medical model.*[69,77] Depression and other psychiatric disorders are medical syndromes, in fact more debilitating than many other chronic medical illnesses, and they result from a stress-diathesis model. The etiology of psychiatric disorders remains unknown, but they clearly involve the complex interaction of genetic or epigenetic vulnerability and environmental stressors. Some stressors are worse than others, and some people are more susceptible to developing a particular syndrome under stress.

No one wants to be depressed or anxious, and it's not the patient's fault. Yet patients frequently blame themselves, guilt being a frequent symptom of depression. Others in their environment, not understanding what patients are going through, may blame them as well. The IPT approach is no-fault, blame-free, shifting negative responsibility from the patient in two ways: by defining guilt and self-criticism as depressive symptoms and by blaming the contextual interpersonal situation (e.g., the troubled marriage or difficult husband) or the depressive disorder itself ("That's the depression talking"). An important, explicit part of IPT involves giving the patient the *sick role,*[7,77] relieving the patient of blame for being ill or having symptoms and conferring the responsibility of working *as* a patient to recover in the time-limited treatment.

A key aspect of the sick role is that the patient has a *treatable condition,* no matter how helpless or hopeless its symptoms may make the patient feel. The therapist also encourages the patient to become expert on depression and the many ways it can be successfully treated.

THE THREE PHASES OF IPT

Opening Phase

The initial phase of IPT lasts a maximum of three sessions, less if efficiency allows (Table 3.1). Its goals are to

1. Collect a history.
2. Set the framework for the treatment to follow.
3. Build a treatment alliance.
4. Begin symptomatic relief.

Table 3.1 TASKS OF THE OPENING PHASE

Steps of Opening Phase	Tasks
1. Taking the history	a. Collect Interpersonal inventory b. Determine diagnosis c. Determine interpersonal problem area (focus)
2. Setting the framework	a. Time limit b. Sick role c. Formulation d. Focus on connection between feelings and events e. "Live dangerously!"
3. Building a treatment alliance	a. Empathic stance b. Respect for autonomy c. Interpersonal context makes sense to patients
4. Symptomatic relief	Follows from the above

TAKING THE HISTORY

In taking a history, the therapist obtains the patient's chief complaint and asks open-ended questions at first, followed by more pointed probes to get details, exploring the patient's current difficulties and his or her understanding of them. The history of present illness should determine when symptoms started and worsened, what the symptoms are, and their interpersonal context. It is often helpful to construct (at least in one's mind) a timeline of the relationship between life events and symptom onset. The difference between taking a history for IPT and for other kinds of therapy lies in the context: you are seeking not only what diagnosis or diagnoses have emerged, but also what might constitute a current interpersonal crisis to work on, and who the patient is as a social animal.

- How does the patient interact with family, friends, work colleagues?
- What patterns recur in relationships?
- How close does the patient get to other people? How willing is he or she to confide feelings to others?
- How comfortable is the patient (not only at present, when comfort is likely to be minimal, but at other times) in asserting himself or herself? In setting limits and fighting with other people?
- How does the patient tolerate and deal with strong emotion?

Gathering this information is part of collecting an *interpersonal inventory*, which is an informal catalogue of the patient's relationships, particularly current relationships. These are the people in the patient's environment who can potentially provide social support, or who may instead be impinging on the patient's comfort (what we term a "role dispute"). After a session or two the therapist should have developed a sense of how populated the patient's world is and how securely attached the patient is in it: how much trust the patient has in others.

Take names: if a patient keeps using pronouns rather than naming significant others, it suggests emotional distancing and intellectualization. Dr. Myrna Weissman, who developed IPT with the late Dr. Gerry Klerman, always talks in her supervision of psychiatric residents about getting to the "nitty gritty" details that bring narratives to life. Insofar as the history will include the pandemic (or other disaster) and the social distancing that has stretched interpersonal bonds, it's important to help the patient see the role that this circumstance may play in why he or she may be feeling so uncomfortable.

Understanding the patient's formative years has importance: Who was the patient in the family sibling order? Whom was he or she closest to growing up? Were there any childhood traumas? What was the atmosphere like in the house: how warm were people with one another, and how did they handle disagreements? (What kind of attachment style might this have bred?) Did the patient make and maintain friendships? What was dating like? While the answers to these questions provide important background, the IPT focus is on current relationships.

A good history of course explores family psychiatric history and the patient's past psychiatric history including prior episodes, traumas, assessment of suicide and violence risk, and response to prior treatments. It's particularly interesting to know how the patient got along with prior therapists, what the patient liked and didn't like about past treatment, and whether the patient felt comfortable raising discomforts or complaints about therapist or therapy. This again reveals some measure of interpersonal comfort and assertiveness. The IPT therapist should invite criticism: "If there's anything I do that bothers you, it won't be intentional; but please bring it up. I want to know how you feel. The first rule of therapy is that you can criticize the therapist."

ORGANIZING THE TREATMENT

Taking a careful history should yield one or more psychiatric diagnoses. Diagnosis is crucial, inasmuch as the diagnostic picture determines what treatments may be appropriate. At the same time, assembling the interpersonal inventory should lead to determination of a treatment focus. In IPT this is fairly straightforward. For patients in the midst or aftermath of a disaster, there are really only three choices, each a psychosocial situation of known depressive risk:[7,69]

(1) *Complicated bereavement.* The death of a significant other—a family member, close friend, or coworker—generally ranks as one of the most stressful of life events. Bereavement evokes powerful feelings, including sadness (grieving the loss), anger (if the death feels unjust, or if the patient resented the deceased), and anxiety (insofar as the death affects the patient's future, e.g., the death of the family breadwinner). Bereavement is often painful, can persist for an extended period, and can mimic many of the feelings and symptoms of depression; but it's normal. Grief is *not* considered pathological unless the individual develops

symptoms such as severe unwarranted guilt and suicidality, at which point it becomes *complicated bereavement*, a subtype of depression.

An unfortunate consequence of disaster is that people die, leaving their survivors to mourn and, in some cases, to develop complicated bereavement or major depression. The current pandemic, in killing extraordinary numbers of citizens, leaves behind hosts of mourners who, if unable to process the painful affects of mourning, may develop complicated bereavement. While we usually think of death as triggering major depression, individuals who witness violent or traumatic deaths, such as frontline medical personnel, may develop PTSD instead of, or in addition to, depression.

(2) *Role dispute.* Good relationships require the ability of both partners to assert their needs and dislikes, to listen to one another, and through this communication to arrive at mutually acceptable compromise. Relationships that lack this process tend to become one-sided, with one partner having his or her needs met, the other not. IPT terms such situations *role disputes*. Imbalanced relationships tend to breed resentment and resignation and can trigger mood and anxiety disorders in vulnerable individuals who are on the losing end of these lopsided relationships. Conversely, anxiety, mood, and trauma-based disorders tend to strain relationships to the patient's disadvantage. Depressed patients famously put the needs of others before their own lest they be rejected, appear selfish, etc. Anxiety generally inhibits confrontation and self-assertion.

Stressors can magnify latent relationship difficulties (see the case of Ms. H in Chapter 7 of this book). A prolonged disaster such as the Covid-19 outbreak, with its huge social consequences, can profoundly affect relationships. Facing the disruption of the pandemic (Table 3.1), individuals may not receive needed social support from others. Joint confinement at close quarters in a crowded household can breed resentment and emotional distance. Living alone during lockdown can intensify feelings of isolation and loneliness. Such strains on relationships can produce symptoms and psychiatric syndromes in vulnerable individuals.

(3) *Role transition.* Most of us don't love change even when it's a positive change, and certainly not when it's a negative one. Too much change can feel like chaos: people feel they're in freefall, their lives out of control. Such environmental stress can trigger psychiatric syndromes in vulnerable individuals. Any major life change that yields the perception of loss of one's anticipated life trajectory may lead to major depression or other disorders: changes like getting married, getting divorced, getting or losing a job, gaining a promotion or being demoted, developing a medical illness. IPT defines these changes as *role transitions*. (The death of a significant other is a special life change. Because of its irrevocability, its separate body of psychosocial evidence, and its slightly different

treatment strategy, IPT separates it as *complicated bereavement* rather than terming it a *role transition*.)

Clearly the pandemic itself is a global, manifold, multifaceted role transition, disrupting life at all levels and likely to be poorly tolerated by anyone appearing in your virtual office.

(4) IPT traditionally has a fourth interpersonal problem area, entitled *interpersonal deficits*. This focal area has several difficulties, beginning with its name, which can sound like a personality disorder. IPT is a life event-focused therapy, and this problem area constitutes something of a residual category for the minority of patients who present without one: that is, with no grief, role dispute, or role transition to work on. These patients are the most isolated to begin with, suffering in effect from loneliness or interpersonal sensitivity. The absence of a life event robs the category of some of its rationale for IPT: the therapist otherwise can point to a life crisis as an explanation for symptoms. The interpersonal deficits category has typically been the hardest category of IPT areas to treat, and we avoid it if we can find any life event to relate to the patient's psychiatric episode. Because a disaster perforce provides a life event, just about any patient presenting in the context of disaster can be treated as having a role transition instead.

Choosing a Problem Area and Giving the Formulation

By the third session, if not before, the IPT therapist has gathered sufficient information to (1) make a psychiatric diagnosis and (2) determine the interpersonal problem area with which to link it.

(1) Not all diagnoses are appropriate for IPT: for example, it has never been tested for but is unlikely to benefit patients with psychosis or with obsessive-compulsive disorder. Nor has IPT fared well as a primary treatment for substance use disorders. On the other hand, most of the likely diagnostic consequences of disaster for which IPT has been shown to work do apply: mood, trauma-related, and anxiety disorders.

It's helpful to *serially measure symptoms* of the target disorder at regular intervals, at the very least at the start, the midpoint, and end of acute treatment. This allows you and the patient to gauge your progress. Instruments might include the Hamilton Depression Rating Scale (Ham-D)[78] or Beck Depression Inventory[79] for depression, the Clinician-Rated PTSD Scale (CAPS-5)[80] or PTSD Checklist (PCL-5)[81] for PTSD, or the Hamilton Anxiety Rating Scale (Ham-A)[82] for anxiety. Getting concrete feedback that scores are improving is remoralizing for patients.

(2) A patient may present with more than one possible interpersonal focus, but for the purposes of a focused, time-limited therapy, it is best to choose a single theme as a way of organizing a likely disorganized

patient. If no one has died, that eliminates the grief/complicated bereavement option. Role transitions and role disputes frequently accompany one another: a change in role is likely to have interpersonal consequences in relationships. For example, a work promotion is a role transition, consequences of which may include altered relationships, and hence disputes, with those around one: having to supervise former colleagues or having less time at home with one's family. It is best to choose a role dispute if there is a key relationship dispute such as a marital crisis and instead to focus on the transition if no one particular relationship problem is prominent. The goal is to maximize the plausibility of the framework for the patient. Whichever area you pick, the same general IPT approach will apply.

Once having established a diagnosis (e.g., major depression) and an interpersonal focus, the therapist presents a *formulation* that links the two, providing the framework for the treatment to follow.[7,83] This feature of IPT organizes the treatment for patient and therapist. The formulation should be as terse as possible, jargon-free, and personalized:

"You've given me a lot of information; please tell me whether I understand what's been going on. As I understand it, you've been vulnerable to depression in the past, and you've become depressed again as the pressures of the Covid pandemic have hit you. Your Hamilton Depression Rating Scale score is 26, which is quite high, in the severe range, but even though you're feeling hopeless from the depression, you in fact have an excellent chance of getting better again and getting your score down into single digits.

"The Covid outbreak has really affected your life and your mood. Your father got sick with the virus, you were worried he might die, and he's had a very slow and difficult course of recovery. You were furloughed from your job, leaving you anxious and a little hopeless about how to take care of your family. And while you've tried to pitch in at home, it's become a little overwhelming and tempers have frayed as you've spent months locked down with your wife and the kids. One on top of the other, these stresses have been overwhelming, and you've been feeling like your life is in chaos, in freefall. It's no wonder you've found this depressing. . . . Is that right?"

If the patient agrees (if the patient does not, listen to the patient's version), continue:

"What may feel like chaos is what we call a 'role transition.' It's hard to go through changes like this, but if you can come to terms with what you've lost and see some of the potentials for your current situation—it's hard when you're depressed, but there generally are positive things you can do—you are likely to improve your life situation, and with it your mood. I suggest that we use the remaining nine sessions of our treatment to work on that.

"Does that make sense to you?"

Alternatively, the formulation might link symptoms to the death of a significant other:

"... losing your partner to Covid sounds like it's been an awful, overwhelming experience that you've struggled to come to terms with—and no wonder. You really miss her, and it's been hard to have a normal mourning and to get the support you need because of the lockdown. We call this 'complicated bereavement,' which is a long-recognized kind of depression. I suggest we spend the remaining ten weeks of therapy helping you to deal with the over-powering feelings you've been struggling to avoid ..."

Or

"... You started to get depressed when your marriage got out of hand, when you and your partner were locked at home together. And, as if things weren't already depressing enough, he began to drink more and to threaten and in-timidate you and the kids, and it's really begun to feel like there's no way out. We call this kind of marital difficulty a 'role dispute,' and it often can bring on depression when someone you count on for support in a crisis turns out to be part of the problem. I suggest we spend the remaining ten sessions helping you figure out how to handle the relationship, which from what you say has also been pretty good over the years, and perhaps can be again. If you can fix the relationship, not only will that improve your situation, but it should also improve your mood symptoms. Does that make sense?"

Whether the life events trigger the depressive episode or follow from it does not matter. The therapist just wants the patient to see that the life circumstance and the mood disorder are connected and that if the patient can solve the inter-personal crisis in his or her environment, it will improve symptoms as well. Nor does a patient beset by multiple pressures in a highly stressful time need to solve everything that's going wrong. Solving one crisis tends to mean gaining new social skills, demonstrating some mastery over the environment, and thus remoralizing the patient within the brief course of acute IPT. If other problems remain, the pa-tient will be less symptomatic, and better skilled and prepared to address them.

The formulation is an important feature of IPT. It explicitly organizes the treat-ment for a potentially distractible patient. It provides an interpersonal goal for the patient to achieve, with the enticement that doing so will both improve the patient's actual life and relieve impairing, painful symptoms. The therapist obtains the patient's explicit agreement on the problem area (e.g., role dispute), which then becomes the focus of treatment. Thereafter, if the therapy should threaten to veer off in another direction, the therapist can acknowledge that this digression sounds interesting, but that only X sessions remain in treatment and that they had agreed to focus on resolving the problem area. The problem area usually makes eminent sense to both therapist and patient, and it is rare for a patient to disagree with a formulation. If that happens, however, the therapist respects the patient's autonomy and negotiates an alternative focus as appropriate, providing a model for adaptive interpersonal interaction.

SETTING THE FRAMEWORK

Giving the patient a formulation is part of setting a treatment framework, and the patient's agreement on this goal marks transition into the middle phase of treatment. Other ground rules that need definition in the initial phase include setting a time limit, providing the sick role, and explaining the general IPT approach.

How to mobilize a patient paralyzed by depression or anxiety is a common psychotherapeutic issue. The IPT *time limit* provides one solution to this problem. In a treatment that does not assign homework, the time limit—generally twelve sessions in as many weeks for major depression; fourteen for PTSD, panic disorder, or social anxiety disorder—pressures the patient to work quickly to resolve his or her life crisis. The absence of homework means that the patient cannot fail to do the homework, which presents a problem in behavioral therapies and leaves the patient feeling like a bad patient. Most patients do not believe they can improve in a matter of weeks (hopelessness is a depressive symptom, helplessness an anxious one), so setting the goal creates some pressure. The patient can move at his or her own pace but knows the clock is ticking. I consider the time limit one of the active strategies that pushes IPT (and IPT patients) forward.

Giving the patient the *sick role*, tailored to the patient's symptoms, temporarily excuses the patient from having to do things that feel too overwhelming.

"You are suffering from depression [or panic disorder, PTSD, etc.], and that makes it much harder to do things. Your energy level is low, you're tired and lack initiative; you feel hopeless about your life. When you're depressed, doing anything is an uphill battle. Think about having a heart condition, or the flu—or, for that matter, Covid-19: you'd give yourself a break for being sick. The reason you don't is partly that depression makes you feel guilty and weak. It's important to understand that major depression is more debilitating than many other medical conditions, and that at least at the start, it's going to be harder to get things done. If there are things you can't do right now because you're depressed, *don't blame yourself: blame the depression.* At the same time, it's important to do what you can to help yourself get better."

This shifting of blame from the patient to the disorder helps to make the symptoms ego-alien and to relieve the patient of guilt. Meanwhile, the time limit (and often the patient's guilt level) helps to ensure that even with this dispensation, the patient will continue to take measures to get better.

To further that process, the therapist outlines the general theme of treatment:

"We're going to focus on the connection between how you're feeling and what's happening in your life. The better you understand that connection, the better you can figure out how to respond to your situation and handle it better. Also, even though you're feeling frightened right now, I'm going to encourage you to 'live dangerously'—not truly dangerously, but to take risks with your feelings and with other people that may stretch your level of comfort right now but can turn out to make a big difference."

Such dangerous living might include expressing one's needs, confronting someone else's unpleasant behavior, or confiding in others, for example.

Again, as part of giving the sick role, it's important to remind the patient:

"Depression is a treatable condition, and it's not your fault. You may feel hopeless, but that's just a depressive symptom. It may be hard to see now, but you have an excellent chance of getting better."

I like to tell patients that as a psychiatrist, I am hopeful when treating someone with anxiety, depression, or PTSD—a diagnosis like schizophrenia is harder to treat.

BUILDING THE TREATMENT ALLIANCE

No treatment, no matter how potent, works unless the therapist can build a sufficient alliance to encourage the patient to accept the treatment. A therapeutic alliance is not only necessary (including for pharmacotherapy[84]) but also contributes to its benefits, instilling a therapeutic trust and accounting for the general placebo effect. Part of the alliance stems from the plausibility of IPT treatment itself and its lack of evident adverse aspects (e.g., no homework, no systematic exposure). But a therapy is in the end only as good as its practitioner, so the IPT therapist's stance is important as well.

As a therapist, take a supportive, empathic role, listening carefully. You don't want to be stiff and formal, nor so relaxed that you invite boundary problems, distract things from the patient's problems to yourself, or seem uncaring. Provide direction only as necessary, in order to encourage the patient's autonomy. In keeping with the IPT medical model, be careful not to criticize the patient, but look to blame the patient's disorder and/or environment for problems that arise. Recognize that the patient is suffering and, even if in some cases difficult to interact with at moments, is struggling to function. For the most part, victims of disaster are highly sympathetic.

An important aspect of IPT—and of any affect-focused therapy, and perhaps any good therapy—is the *tolerance of affect*.[85] It's important to elicit the strong emotions that sit at the heart of mood, anxiety, and trauma syndromes, feelings that patients fear and try to avoid. One of our helpful interventions in adapting IPT for PTSD was the suggestion that "feelings are powerful but not dangerous."[3] If a patient can sit with an emotion rather than avoiding it, it may be tiring and upsetting, but the surge of feeling informs the patient about something important in his or her life, and after a time it subsides and becomes less of a problem to deal with in future. (This is a principle of behavioral exposure therapy.)

So it's important to evoke feelings, to normalize them (aside from those that you can label as symptoms), and to resist the temptation to rush in and reassure patients. As treatment progresses, the patient generally comes to realize that feelings are tolerable and even interpersonally informative. As we told benumbed PTSD patients who were suppressing their "dangerous" emotions, it's better to know how you feel even if the feelings are painful: without knowing how you feel, you're flying blind in the interpersonal world, and it's impossible to know whom to trust.[3]

Your role is also to *model* for the patient that feelings are tolerable, not dangerous. It's unhelpful to be too chipper or cheery with a suffering patient. Acknowledge their pain; don't dismiss it, explore it. Silence can be productive if you're both attuned to the patient's strong emotion. Show the patient it's not dangerous. Your face can reflect the painful emotion. If you instead change the subject to some less affect-laden topic, or if you provide immediate reassurance, the patient may feel you misunderstand, fear, or are trivializing the relevant situation and feelings—contradicting the message of IPT that feelings are not dangerous.

Thus in approaching the patient's anxiety, depression, or PTSD (and the feelings these evoke in you), you want to communicate to the patient your recognition that it's awful to experience these symptoms, and they have something to do with the life circumstance in which the patient is struggling. Empathize at points (and not too quickly, which cuts off exploration) that it must feel awful. You and the patient can both sit with these feelings, to understand them, to show that they're not so toxic. And then—again, not too soon—you can point out that the patient has a treatable disorder, that even if he or she feels hopeless, that's a symptom and not an accurate prognosis.

In short, the therapeutic stance in IPT is serious (recognizing the patient's suffering), sympathetic, patient, and ultimately (but not prematurely) optimistic: the illness is treatable, and you have confidence in the patient's ability to navigate through this difficult time. Acting as this kind of supportive ally strengthens the alliance. All of this takes places within the life event-focused treatment structure that the IPT framework provides.

Psychoeducation can be helpful but is best limited to small bites. Patients don't like to be lectured to, and any understanding they gain from an extended speech is likely to be an intellectualization rather than the emotional experience that cements understanding. (Recall that most people who attend an hour-long lecture remember at most one or two ideas.) The most useful psychoeducation comes in the previously described scenario, after the patient has been experiencing symptoms or tolerating feelings in the session: as a clarification in an emotional context, not as a standalone, abstract explanation. It usually involves reifying the target diagnosis as a medical illness, providing the sick role: "That's the depression talking"; "It's possible to have mixed feelings"; "The people you're closest to can be the ones you hate the most when they let you down"; "When you've been through something that awful and upsetting, of course you're going to have very upsetting feelings."

Anxious and depressed patients often feel helpless and hopeless and may ask you what to do. Again, don't succumb to temptation. The patient may actually understand the situation in question better than you do. Furthermore, you want to increase the patient's sense of competence and autonomy. Even if you give good advice, the patient takes it, and it works, the patient will conclude: "Lucky I have a good therapist. I never would have come up with that on my own, I'm an incapable idiot." So much better to put the ball back in the patient's court: "What options do you have?" is an important IPT intervention.[7] The patient will often come up with things you might not have thought of, but even if you had, it's better that it comes from the patient. If that probe doesn't suffice, go further: "What have you tried so far?" Explore what has worked, what hasn't, and whether the patient's efforts have been thwarted by depressive symptoms. In the course of this discussion, the patient may generate other options. Always treat the patient as a capable individual, even if the patient doesn't feel like one.

The initial phase of IPT is kept brief to allow ample time for the subsequent phases, but it sets the stage for everything that follows. As this chapter suggests, it requires the therapist to complete numerous tasks. Yet these fairly basic steps—taking a history, setting a framework, and building a treatment alliance—are powerful and organizing. They provide a helpful structure, which patients in or after a disaster sorely need. They provide hope in the form of a plausible treatment approach that explains the patient's current suffering in the context of a *treatable illness, arising in the context of external stressors, that is not the patient's fault*, with a therapist who is understanding, recognizes the patient's suffering, and yet conveys hope for improvement in what may seem an impossibly short (but research-proven) time frame.

Middle Phase

Once the patient has accepted the formulation, treatment moves to the middle phase, where the bulk of the work takes place. We will cover the middle phase in the next chapter.

Termination Phase

The last few sessions of time-limited treatment continue the themes of earlier weeks but also address the fact that therapy (or at least acute weekly therapy) is approaching its end. Often the patient is feeling much better, but hasn't been feeling better long enough to fully trust that it will last. The patient's confidence may still be shaky, and he or she may worry about residual symptoms or fear a relapse. Goals of the termination phase (Chapter 8 of this book) include integrating gains, acknowledging feelings about therapy ending, and looking ahead to future problems.

- *Looking back at the treatment.* If the patient is feeling better, as most IPT patients will, it's important to place credit where it's due. Patients are often grateful to and attribute their gains to the therapist, but that's neither fair nor helpful. Reviewing what has happened in therapy is helpful to underscore and help the patient integrate what has happened, and what he or she has achieved.

  Review the change in rating scale scores, remark on the improvement ("That's great!"), and ask: "*Why* are you feeling so much better?" The answer relates to what the patient has accomplished in a matter of weeks, and while feeling awful, to resolve the interpersonal problem area that has been the focus of treatment. Although you as the therapist may have been helpful and encouraging, it's the patient who did the hard work in his or her real life and has made concrete changes. In the process, the patient may have acquired new social skills (better self-assertion; learning how to fight back and renegotiate a role dispute) and mobilized social support, expanding his or her daily activities in a productive way, and hopefully has acquired a greater sense of control over both internal feelings and external relationships. This review itself generally bolsters patient's self-confidence and provides an opportunity to reinforce new social skills.

- *Looking at the present.* If the patient does not raise the issue of termination spontaneously, you can say:

"We only have a few sessions left, we're approaching the end of our treatment. How are you feeling about our stopping three weeks from now?"

Part of a good relationship involves ending it well. Terminating a relationship is a role transition and a loss; the patient may have positive and negative feelings about the treatment experience and the relationship he or she has had with you. IPT generally encourages patients to recognize their feelings as healthy interpersonal guides and to verbalize them when appropriate. For depressed patients, distinguishing the sadness of separation from the too-close-for-comfort feeling of depression is often useful. As an IPT therapist, it's also appropriate to tell a patient at the end of therapy:

"It's been a pleasure working with you, impressive to see you take control of your life and your symptoms and to make so many changes in just a few weeks. You've done a great job, and I'm going to miss working with you."

But don't lead with that. Wait to hear what the patient has to say.

- *Looking ahead.* Termination should involve anticipating future problems as well. What clouds lie on the horizon? What interpersonal problems can the patient foresee, and how can he or she deal with them? The skills the patient has used to solve the interpersonal focus of the current episode may apply, and you can role play these.

If the patient has not improved in the time-limited interval of IPT, that too needs to be acknowledged. It does not make clinical sense to perpetuate a treatment that has not yielded benefit after several months when effective treatment alternatives exist. Patients who don't improve, or improve insufficiently, tend to blame themselves, and that's not helpful. You can remind the patient that *no treatment works for everyone,* and—much as you might do if an antidepressant medication hadn't worked—blame the treatment approach and raise alternatives. The most important outcome is that the patient not be too discouraged to explore other treatment options that might well help.[86] This might include pharmacotherapy, CBT, evidence-based psychodynamic therapy, or some other approach as clinically indicated.

CONTINUATION/MAINTENANCE IPT

Some patients may have shown partial benefit in IPT—say, 30% to 50% improvement—but remain symptomatic, perhaps in part due to continuing stressors of the ongoing disaster. The patient's Ham-D score may have fallen from 28 to 15: a meaningful and impressive improvement, no longer severely depressed, but still in the moderately depressed range. If so, continuation IPT may be appropriate. The same applies to patients who have achieved recovery (Ham-D ≤7) but face a high risk of relapse or recurrence without maintenance therapy. If so, it's still important to terminate acute treatment at the end of the original time frame, presenting the rationale for continuing treatment, and then recontract for ongoing IPT, perhaps for six months or a year or two.

Maintenance IPT has been shown to benefit acute IPT responders and to protect against future depressive episodes.[75,76,87] The maintenance phase allows a shift from the original interpersonal focus to deal with changing situations and to change session frequency as needed. You and the patient might agree to continue weekly therapy or to meet biweekly or even monthly—doses at which maintenance IPT has been tested.[75,76,87]

ADAPTATIONS FOR DISASTER

The rationale for this book is that we are facing an ongoing global disaster with ongoing psychiatric consequences. Adapting IPT for this extended interval requires coming to terms with problematic aspects of these times. It is hard to predict the future. (Who could have foreseen this pandemic and its concatenations?) I hope against hope that by the date of publication social distancing has diminished and people are able to safely return to more regular schedules, in which case some of

Table 3.2 DISASTER ADAPTATIONS

Problem	Intervention
Covid-19 pandemic	Acknowledge the crisis
Collapse of routine	Adjust social zeitgebers: Sleep schedule Exercise schedule Activities schedule
Isolation: loss of social contacts	Encourage maintenance of social connections and supports
Excessive social media use	Ask about extent of use Limit social media exposure

the following suggestions (Table 3.2) may have less urgency. The clinician reader can employ them flexibly.

Acknowledging the Crisis

The first step is to contextualize the patient in the pandemic crisis. These are no ordinary times, the patient is under no ordinary pressures, and such stressors take a toll. The general IPT formula is, "You've had to deal with so much, no wonder you're feeling depressed. It's hard, you're suffering, but there are things you can do to get yourself out of this." Rarely can this have been truer.

Adjusting Social Zeitgebers

As discussed in Chapter 1 of this book, one source of distress and disorientation has been the collapse of normal routine. Being homebound and lacking scheduling can scramble one's biological clock, affecting mood, sleep, energy, concentration, and general functioning. The solution is to encourage patients to impose order, to fabricate schedules—however artificial this may seem—to organize and stabilize their days. In presenting this, you can refer to social zeitgeber theory[19] and the need for such "time givers" to anchor our days.

    Some of this phenomenon is physical: a healthy sleep schedule leaves us rested, exercise is invigorating and burns muscle tension. When, some nineteen hundred years ago, the Roman poet Juvenal advocated praying for *mens sana in corpore sano* ("a healthy mind in a healthy body"), he was perhaps intuiting something about biorhythms. Both kinds of health are important, and the two are connected. Thus the general recommendations of sleep hygiene include going to sleep and waking up at the same time every day, in effect conditioning the body to a restful sleep cycle. Limiting stimulation such as television, alcohol, late snacking, and bright light in the evening can help prepare the body for sleep.[88,89] Similarly, regular aerobic exercise a couple of times a week dissipates the physical tension and agitation that result from and reinforce psychic anxiety. Research shows that such exercise (at least in group format) at least temporarily benefits depressive symptoms.[90]

During the lockdown, one of my suddenly homebound depressed patients reported managing to maintain a consistent pace of 23,000 smartphone-recorded steps per day—in his apartment! He found this improved his mood. For many others, taking a brisk walk outdoors or doing an online video workout has been an invigorating relief from the claustrophobia of an apartment.

Beyond the physical, it's good to have things to look forward to on your calendar, rather than to feel bored. This problem has worsened as the lockdown has dragged on: people were officially discouraged from leaving their homes, and even if they did so (which, with appropriate six-foot social distancing, might be healthy), there was little to do. Entertainment and eateries had largely shut down.

Within a daily schedule, it may be useful to plan regular meal times, family time, etc. On a broader scale, most of us have activities we have "saved for a rainy day," a day that may now have arrived. (In fact, we're now well beyond forty days and forty nights.) Scheduling time to do anything productive is likely to feel better than twiddling one's thumbs, playing endless games of solitaire, or engaging in too much social media (see the following discussion). Challenge the patient to make the best possible use of this surfeit of unscheduled time. For patients deluged with childcare, home chores, work, and other responsibilities, help them to carve out time for personal pleasures or initiatives, or even just rest, where possible. In all cases, identify the disruption of social activities and physical rhythms as a symptom-producing risk of the pandemic that the patient can try to address.

Drs. Ellen Frank, Holly Swartz, and others have used interpersonal psychotherapy and social rhythms (IPSRT) techniques to treat patients whose bipolar I[9,15] and bipolar II[91] diagnoses make them exquisitely sensitive to the neurobiological effects of temporal disruption. Their research shows that using the IPSRT Social Rhythm Metric (Table 3.3; https://www.ipsrt.org; there is now even an app) helped bipolar I patients to organize their daily rhythms.[92] Under circumstances of social disruption, these are generally healthy adjustments for everyone.

Minimizing Isolation

"Social distancing" protects against Covid-19 infection but unfortunately puts social support at risk. In the setting of a "shelter in place" lockdown that largely confines non-essential workers to their homes, people may be cut off from important friends, colleagues, and family members. It's important to acknowledge this as an unwanted difficulty of the pandemic that has important social and psychic consequences. Under the circumstances, how can the patient maintain and even expand needed social supports?

In taking an interpersonal inventory, note not only who the significant others are but also where they are located. Are they within walking distance? Biking distance? We are treating patients living in New York City who had family members

Table 3.3 SOCIAL RHYTHM METRIC–II—FIVE-ITEM VERSION (SRM-II-5)

Directions:

- Write the ideal target time you would like to do these daily activities.
- Record the time you activity did the activity each day.
- Record the people involved in the activity: 0 = Others present; 2 = Other activity involved; 3 = Others very stimulating

Date (week of): _____

Activity	Target time	Sunday		Monday		Tuesday		Wednesday		Thursday		Friday		Saturday	
		People	Time	People	Time	People	Time	People	Time	People	Time	People	Time	People	Time
Out of bed															
Start work/school/ volunteer/family care															
Dinner															
To bed															
Rate MOOD each day from –5 to +5: –5 = very depressed +5 = very depressed															

From Treating Bipolar Disorder: A Clinical's Guide to Interpersonal Social Rhythm Therapy by Elton Frank. Copyright 2005 by the Guilford Press. Permission to Photography this appendix is granted to purchasers of this book for personal use only (see copyright page for details).

Appendix I—Social Rhythm Metric—II—Five-Item Version (SRM-II-5) from p. 164 of Treating Bipolar Disorder: A Clinician's Guide to Interpersonal Social Rhythm Therapy by Ellen Frank. Reprinted with permission from Guilford Press.

or lovers in northern New Jersey—a once easily bridgeable distance now rendered impassable by the dangers of public transport. The roughly half of all New Yorkers who relied on the subway stopped using it en masse when Covid-19 hit. Ridership fell by 90%, cutting off Manhattanites from Brooklynites.[93] With understanding of the infectivity of the virus still fragmentary, and with some level of anxiety appropriate depending upon one's risk factors (age, medical status, etc.), friends have been afraid to see each other, even with masks and appropriate six-foot social distancing. So social bonds fray; people feel cut off and isolated. It's a difficult time to develop new relationships or to date.

Under such circumstances, it's important to raise the need for social connection with patients. How can they maintain connections? Are there people they can safely see, outdoors, at arms' length, in person? What about Facetime, Zoom, Skype, and other ways of maintaining contact? Almost any direct connection, voice or video, seems preferable to texting, where affect is so easily lost or prone to misinterpretation. Preserving and enhancing social support is likely to lower symptoms and increase sense of well-being.

Limiting Social Media Use

Staying caught up with news developments is helpful in a time of danger, but too much media use may breed anxiety. Social media may help to diminish social isolation to a degree—depending upon how truly friendly you are with online "friends"—but excessive involvement may mean exposure to misinformation and contagious anxiety. In China during this pandemic, individuals with high social media exposure in an online survey were almost twice as likely to report depressive and anxiety symptoms as those with less social media exposure.[24] Previous studies[25,26] have documented links between excessive social media use and depression,[27,28] anxiety,[28,29] loneliness,[30] and suicidal ideation.[31] This literature has technical limitations, but it does point to a potential problem.

Under the circumstances, it seems appropriate to ask patients about their social media use and to suggest its potential dangers in excess.

From these domains one can construct a "Covid Checklist" to consider (Box 3.2): a series of questions to ask patients to gauge how disruptive the disaster has been and whether the patient is responding appropriately or excessively to the changed situation.

As part of evaluation for treatment, the clinician should always consider whether to combine psychotherapy with pharmacotherapy. For patients with severe and highly chronic symptoms, or high suicide risk, combined treatment may have advantages over monotherapy. Psychotherapy and pharmacotherapy work in different ways, and medication tends to work faster. Faster response might save a patient's life. For major depression, the combination of the two modalities overall has never shown less efficacy than monotherapy,[94] although not all patients will need both. For PTSD and anxiety disorders, there are too few trials to demonstrate this, but the same principle generally applies. The IPT

Box 3.2

THE COVID BEHAVIORAL CHECKLIST: HOW STRESSFUL ARE EFFECTS OF THE DISASTER?

1. *How worried are you about getting infected?*
   a. How exposed are you to possible infection? (High risk? Low risk?)
   b. What precautions are you taking? (Appropriate? Excessive?)
2. *How has the disruption of daily routine affected you?*
   a. How much of a daily schedule do you have these days? (Do you have things to look forward to?)
   b. Are you still working? (Remotely? What's it like? Do you miss your commute?)
   c. How are you sleeping? What's your sleep schedule? How regular is it? Are you generally rising and going to bed at the same time every day?
   d. How often and for how long are you getting out of the house? How much are you exercising?
3. *How much social contact are you having with other people?*
   a. Are you staying in touch with friends and family? Are you actually seeing them?
   b. Are there people you can talk to about how you're feeling?
   c. How is your home situation? (Too crowded and irritating? Too isolated?)
4. *How much time are you spending on social media?* (Hours a day?)

---

medical model presents no conflicts in combining the two modalities: the therapist can compare it to using insulin and a behavioral diet and exercise regimen for diabetes, for instance.

WHAT NOT TO DO

Every psychotherapy session comprises a sequence of therapist/patient interactions where the therapist is likely to recognize a pattern and must decide what to do with it. The therapist's training in different therapies influences such pattern recognition. Thus a CBT therapist may "automatically" identify negative cognitions in speaking with a depressed patient, and a psychodynamically trained therapist may recognize unconscious conflicts and transferential material. The question is what to do with this. The danger exists that a multiply skilled therapist will recognize one element at one point and intervene in CBT fashion, a second element that provokes a psychodynamic intervention, and so on. This is what's called eclectic therapy—a little of this and a little of that—and I will argue that it's not good for several reasons.[86,95,96]

The goal of a brief, time-limited treatment is to provide organization and focus for a disorganized and unfocused patient. To do so, it's important to keep the therapy itself streamlined and organized. One of the beauties of the IPT approach is its thematic simplicity, which an eclectic approach inevitably corrupts. Everything in IPT focuses on the connection between affect and life circumstance; introducing a cognitive or transferential or behavioral element will not fit that paradigm and is a distraction.

If your treatment interventions vary over the course of treatment, even if they are all accurate in, for example, identifying negative automatic thoughts, the patient is likely to think you're a brilliant therapist, you always know what to say, but the patient may not always understand the method you're trying to communicate. A patient is likely to leave a twelve-week treatment much changed, but will probably retain only a few basic pointers. (Think about the answers patients give when you ask them about what was helpful in prior therapies. I have had patients return years after a course of treatment and tell me that what they had found most useful was something I hadn't recalled saying or didn't think was important at all.) Your goal is to give the patient a few interpersonal tools to take away from treatment: trust your feeling, express them to handle encounters, recognize symptoms, mobilize social supports. Patients will be less likely to leave with a clear game plan for the future if the therapy itself has been unclear or too complicated. So pick one therapy and stick to it: if you're going to do IPT, try to do *only* IPT.

4

Life Crises

Grief, Role Disputes, and Role Transitions

Upon agreeing to the IPT formulation, you and the patient enter the middle phase of IPT and focus on the central interpersonal problem area: *grief (complicated bereavement), role dispute,* or *role transition.* Each of these focal problem areas has slightly different but overlapping strategies.[7] Regardless of the problem area, each session after the initial one follows the same general structure and sequence (Table 4.1). (Again, post-disaster patients benefit from structure.)

STARTING SESSIONS

In opening an IPT treatment, you naturally introduce yourself to the patient and elicit a history. In every session after the first one, even if you are still gathering information in the initial phase, the session should have a structure, beginning with its opening. Greet the patient with "How have things been since we last met?"

This simple question helpfully organizes the session that follows. IPT emphasizes the link between mood state and events (see Figure 3.1 in Chapter 3 of this book), and asking this question does so immediately. "Since we last met" requests an interval history. IPT sessions are generally spaced at weekly intervals so that enough time elapses for things to happen in the patient's life, and the treatment focuses on those weekly events and their related feelings. The patient is likely either to relate an event from the prior week ("I had a fight with my partner." "I didn't get the job I interviewed for." "My child was sick.") or a mood. If an upsetting event occurs, express sympathy ("Oh, I'm sorry to hear that"), then ask, "How did that make you feel?" Alternatively, if the patient voices a feeling ("I've been feeling more anxious"; "I've been more depressed"), the reciprocal reply is "I'm sorry to hear that . . . did anything happen that contributed to your feeling worse?"

Thus after two questions, you have helped the patient to identify a recent, affectively charged life circumstance. Ideally this will relate to the interpersonal treatment focus: for example, a recent struggle with the partner in the central role dispute. Even if it does not, it's an opportunity for the patient to recognize the

Table 4.1 SEQUENCE OF IPT SESSIONS

Maneuver	Goal/Outcome
Opening question	Link mood and event
Explore recent affectively-charged event	Reconstruct event with blow-by-blow Interactions Patient's feelings Whether patient verbalized feelings
Elicit emotions	How did it feel? Reasonable reactions? → Normalize emotions
Evaluate outcome	Did patient accomplish what he or she wanted? What went right or wrong? (Communication analysis) How did patient feel afterward?
Explore options	If things went poorly, what other options exist? Role play

connection between feeling state and life context. Moreover, this recent, emotionally evocative incident often provides an excellent opportunity for understanding how the patient interacts with others, and where his or her syndrome may be impairing interpersonal functioning.

The next step is to reconstruct this recent event. What happened? What was the patient expecting? The goal here is to elicit a blow-by-blow transcript of whatever occurred: what the patient said, what the other person said, what the patient then felt, how the patient responded, what the patient said then, etc. "How did you feel then?" And then what happened?" . . . "And then how did you feel?" "What did you say?" . . . "And then what happened?"

Patients generally have an easier time relating the events (although when too emotionally charged, these can get disorganized) than the feelings they had, but it's equally important to understand those moment to moment emotional responses.

THERAPIST: . . . I'm sorry to hear it. Can you tell me what happened?
PATIENT: Well, you know, you and I had been talking about my talking to my husband, so I tried. I said, "Did you read that book about depression I'd asked you to look at?" And he said, "No, it looked too long." And he went back to reading the newspaper. And that was about it. We haven't really talked since.
THERAPIST: Hmm. How did you feel when he said that?
PATIENT: It was pretty much what I expected.
THERAPIST: Yes, you had had your doubts about how much he would respond. But surely you had some feeling when he said that?
PATIENT: No. Not really. . . . well, I guess I was a tiny bit disappointed.
THERAPIST: Yes?

PATIENT: A little disappointed. But I don't like to burden him, and we have a good marriage, but I wasn't expecting much.

THERAPIST: Just a little disappointed?

PATIENT: Well, disappointed.

THERAPIST: Why?

PATIENT: I guess, he knows I'm depressed and I guess I was hoping he cared enough to check into what I'm going through. So yes, I guess that hurt my feelings.

THERAPIST: Is it reasonable to feel hurt and disappointed if you ask him to do something that has meaning for you, and he doesn't?

PATIENT: Yes, I think so. It's not like he doesn't read long books, and *Darkness Visible* isn't even very long.

THERAPIST: Good point. . . . Did you have any other feelings after he said that?

PATIENT: No. . . . well, maybe I was a little frustrated.

This vignette hopefully illustrates some of the simple elegance of an IPT session. It instantly focuses the patient on a recent interpersonal encounter and explores the patient's behavior and emotional reactions during that interchange. Even this very brief story reveals a lot. First, it really does sound like there is a role dispute in the marriage. The depressed wife, who has been loath to burden her husband by asking him for anything on her own behalf—depressed patients generally being much more focused on the needs of others than on their own—has ventured a request relating to her own mental health, and the husband casually dismisses it. The patient is not really attuned to her feelings in the moment. The marital encounter ends there, too: there is no further discussion. A more assertive (less depressed) marital partner might have persisted: "This is important to me. I wanted to help you understand what I'm going through, and I'm hurt and disappointed and angry that you just ignore me the one time I ask you for help." One hopes such a moment might arise further along in treatment.

Figuring out what happened in such an encounter is, in IPT terminology, *communication analysis*. What can the patient take away from such an incident? How does he or she understand the interchange? What is the patient's understanding of his or her own wishes, feelings, and intentions, and the complementary wishes, feelings, intentions, and motives of the other person? How much time to devote to such discussion will vary from session to session and patient to patient and constitutes a clinical choice. (If this is session 2, you may want to move from this episode back to history gathering.) The goals are to broaden the patient's understanding of such encounters, increase tolerance of confrontations—"confrontation" sounds like trouble to many patients, but can be necessary and helpful for adjusting relationships—and to increase emotional reflection on such issues. This is a point at which IPT overlaps with mentalization.[95]

ELICITING AFFECT

Although the principal goal of IPT is to relieve symptoms, one of its great side benefits is the opportunity to develop a broader emotional vocabulary. Patients with panic disorder are often oddly detached from their emotions (which is why panic attacks seem to hit them "out of the blue," despite their usually clear connection to some interpersonal incident[97]), and patients with PTSD seem to consciously suppress them.[3,5] Depressed patients often see negative affects as part of their "badness," a reason people don't like them.[7] Thus many patients, when asked, may minimize negative affects, or at most concede, "I was a little upset." That's a start, but we really want patients to identify their feelings more specifically, inasmuch as different kinds of "upset" have different meanings. Many people do not recognize such distinctions, yet the distinctions are crucial. Very broadly, anxiety signals a potential environmental threat; sadness signals loss; anger signals mistreatment or injustice.

So if a patient says he or she is "upset," ask: "What kind of 'upset'?" Let the patient think about this for a while. Some patients will volunteer cognitions or report actions rather than emotions: "I was trying to get this done"; "I got busy." Most patients who are uncomfortable with anger will at best acknowledge disappointment or hurt or at most a little frustration or annoyance—"angry" or "mad" sounding too frightening as responses. It's best not to spoon-feed options to patients, who may simply process them intellectually. Better to engage the patient in re-creation of a real-life encounter and probe the reactions there, helping the patient to understand these emotions in the moment, in context.

Patients frequently struggle with the concept that any event may evoke multiple and conflicting emotions. Some will find it easier to get angry at strangers than at more significant others on whom they depend. A sleep-deprived, depressed mother whose baby has been screaming all night may feel like a horrible person for wanting to throw the infant out the window—not that she would ever do such a thing, but even the thought or impulse reveals just how awful she really is. Yet *it's often the people we really love whom we can also really hate when they frustrate or disappoint us.* (And where is her husband while she's up all night caring for the infant?) Helping patients to recognize their feelings, to interpret them as signals in an interpersonal situation (I can love my baby and be angry at her, too, and love my husband but resent that he's sleeping while I'm kept awake) opens another dimension of understanding for patients and helps to normalize them.

When a patient reports a disappointing encounter, reinforce the patient's affective responses to it. Acknowledge the disappointment that it went poorly and give the patient credit for at least trying despite feeling so badly already. In short, validate the feelings as normal, informative responses to the situation. Then the next step is to figure out what went wrong and how the patient could respond to that situation (which is often likely to recur in one form or another) in future. "What options do you have [for handling it differently]?" Anxious, depressed, and discouraged patients often initially see no options, but one of the points of

IPT is that *there are always things you can do*. Options may be difficult, or limited, but they exist and may be worth trying; it's the patient's symptoms that obscure or discourage such choices. To respect the patient's autonomy, put the question to the patient rather than offering suggestions. With a little gentle prodding (silent expectation; "What have you tried in the past?"), patients often come up with ideas.

The patient's emotional response to the recent encounter frequently provides a pathway to recognizing options. Part of the reason to normalize painful affects for patients is to relieve the pain these "bad" feelings cause them. More important, though, is that normalizing anger or sadness or anxiety may lead to the patient accepting and finding a way to verbalize these feelings to others. Telling a third party how she feels ("Sometimes my baby gets me so angry at night when she won't sleep and won't let me sleep—even though I love her to pieces") might provide social support. More directly, feeling justified to have a discussion with the better-rested husband might lead to a more equitable child care and sleeping arrangement, decreasing resentment and easing the patient's interactions with both baby and husband.

Having a concept for action is one thing, really planning to do it another. For patients who struggle with self-assertion or communicating their feelings, as most anxious, depressed, and traumatized patients do, practice is essential. Hence once you and the patient have agreed on an option ("Good idea," crediting the patient for having come up with it), it is important to role play the encounter, often several times. This gives the patient as well as the therapist a chance to evaluate:

(1) *Content*: Is the patient saying what he or she wants to say? Is there a direct and clear request for action? ("I need your help in handling Sascha's sleeping schedule. I just can't do it all myself.") Is it phrased as a question or a declarative statement? (There's a big difference between, "Could you maybe help?" and "I need you to help.")

Has the patient made any mention of his or her feelings? ("I don't like it when . . ."; "It would really make me happy if . . ."; "You really hurt my feelings when . . ."; "It makes me angry when you. . . .") A request generally carries much more weight when it arrives with an emotional attachment.

(2) *Tone of voice*: If the patient is angry, is that evident from the tone of voice, or does he or she sound timid and frightened? If a patient is anxious, does that come across, or is the patient monotonal and constricted?

To increase the odds of success, it's often helpful to explore contingencies with the patient and to role play these scenarios as well. What does the patient worry might go wrong? Suppose the other party objects? Or gets angry too? (What options does the patient have for responding?) How does the patient anticipate the other person might respond, and how could the patient respond to that? What might be good or bad timing for an encounter? What else could go wrong?

With a little practice, the patient usually gains confidence in asserting needs or dislikes—an often novel step. Discussing such issues, validating the underlying feelings, and building skills through role play primes the patient for eventual action. When that action occurs is up to the patient: you will have prepared the patient for an important encounter, but you should not assign homework. The time pressure of treatment will generally do the rest: the patient knows the clock is ticking.

This is the kind of "living dangerously" that you will have already encouraged the patient to do, to explore and embody feelings to change his or her life. It's good to "live dangerously" and explore options during therapy: if things go well, the patient will feel better; if things go poorly, at least the patient has tried, can review what happened with you, learn from the experience, regroup, and try a different option. Patients will differ in their risk tolerance and their readiness for change.[98] While it can be a little frustrating and anxiety-provoking to observe and wait for weeks before the patient risks the encounter, it's better to leave the timing to the patient, who can also then take independent credit for its success.

Sometimes the patient will try to employ the role-played situation in real life and find it doesn't work. If this occurs, the next session will have a great topic in answer to "How have things been since we last met?" and you can try to figure out what happened. Again, give the patient credit for having tried to fix things, see how you can learn from what went amiss, and explore further options to try to resolve the situation. It takes two people to compromise. If the patient is facing an impossible other, this may become clear with repeated attempts to negotiate a problem. At that point, the patient may recognize that whatever the problem is in the relationship, it's not the patient's fault but the other's intransigence. That shifts the blame, as well as the patient's perspective on the dilemma in which the patient finds himself or herself.

If the patient risks a confrontation or makes an important life change and it goes well, explore the particulars ("How did it go? . . . How did that feel?") but don't shy away from offering congratulations. ("Amazing work!") Such a moment often represents the first real test of a new skill, a step outside of the patient's previous comfort zone—it's a big deal. Beyond whatever specific outcome took place, it's a model for new functioning that deserves reinforcement. Such signal events often are therapeutic turning points, "success experiences"[99] associated with symptom relief. Patients gain at least a tentative grasp of a new skill ("I can ask for a raise and my boss listens to me"; "My spouse and I can have a productive fight and solve something, without the relationship exploding") and gain some sense of mastery over both their emotional life and their interpersonal environment. When, in the termination phase of IPT, you ask a patient *why* he or she is feeling better, moments like this come to mind. In effect, in a kind of shorthand or synecdoche, such victories encapsulate the IPT experience. Underlining the importance of such moments helps patients to incorporate them.

This sequence of IPT sessions should make clear why IPT helps patients to understand their feelings, change their interpersonal environments, build interpersonal skills, and mobilize social support. It's really the whole thrust of the therapy.

Table 4.2 MOOD AND LIFE EVENTS INTERACT AT THREE LEVELS

Level	Structural Interval	Goal
Macro	Overarching treatment	Diagnostic recovery
Micro	Session	Linking mood/circumstance/actions
Underlying	Communication analysis	Improving reflective function

Rather than focusing on cognitions and their evidence, on unconscious conflicts, or on the transference (all issues the IPT therapist may observe but generally does not address), the focus is entirely on mood and real-life situations.

The simple thematic elegance of IPT makes it relatively easy for distressed patients to understand, even when anxiety, depression, or trauma distract their concentration. The interaction of mood and life circumstance (see Figure 3.1 in Chapter 3) is enacted at three parallel levels (Table 4.2). At the broadest level, the connection applies to the time-limited treatment as a whole: the formulation in the initial phase links the symptomatic episode (major depression) to the interpersonal crisis that becomes the treatment focus (role transition of loss of job). In each treatment session, the opening question ("How have things been since we last met?") guides the patient toward recognition of recent life circumstances and their effect on the patient's mood, and vice versa. Finally, in communication analysis dissecting a particular encounter, the patient explores feelings at the blow-by-blow level of a conversational exchange ("How did you feel when he said that?"). This structural consistency surely adds to the coherence and plausibility of the treatment. Maintaining the clarity of this treatment structure is an argument against therapeutic eclecticism.

THE PROBLEM AREAS IN GREATER DETAIL

This section describes the issues and maneuvers that distinguish the three IPT focal problem areas. Diagnosis-specific clinical examples appear in subsequent chapters.

GRIEF (COMPLICATED BEREAVEMENT)

No single life event is generally considered as stressful as the death of a significant other. On scales of life events, death ranks at the top (and the death of one's child at the very top).[100] The death of someone close evokes a host of feelings so strong that societies have developed a host of religious and secular rituals to cushion them. Grief is expectably powerful and persists in varying forms for years. Its expression can overlap with symptoms of depression, such as sleep and appetite disturbance, difficulty enjoying things, and deep sadness. Processing the

emotions and emotional memories that attend grief is not easy, but it is important. Attending a funeral, burial, wake, or shiva evokes these feelings and allows
sharing them with others, enlisting social support. Again: grief is painful but
normal, not psychopathological.

One risk for developing depression in adult life, as Freud noted a century ago
in *Mourning and Melancholia*,[101] is the death of a parent during one's childhood.
Individuals who find the pain of bereavement emotions too threatening tend to
throw themselves into preparing the funeral or catering the wake, keeping themselves too busy to really attend. ("I didn't have time to cry or think about her.")
They may fear that if they start to mourn they'll never stop, or that the strength
of their emotions may shatter them. As a result, they avoid mourning—and end
up depressed, dragging around and trying to minimize intense emotional pain.

The pandemic has complicated this scenario by increasing the number of
deaths (by more than 100,000 Americans, as of late May 2020; over 130,000, by
early July) and complicating the rituals of mourning. Social distancing has effectively blocked in-person religious and funeral services. People have tried to
conduct "virtual" Zoom memorials, which may partially mitigate this but cannot
really replace the social intermingling so crucial to not feeling alone with one's
powerful emotions. Thus we may expect—and are already seeing—many patients
suffering from complicated bereavement.

History

In taking the patient's history and gathering an interpersonal inventory, ascertain
whether anyone has died, as this could become the treatment focus. IPT requires
an actual death for this category; other losses are considered role transitions. If
someone has died, how close was the patient to the deceased? Is there a temporal
connection between the death of the other person and the onset of the patient's
depressive symptoms? Has the patient put away her late husband's belongings, or
has everything been left exactly as it was, as a shrine? The death often feels like a
rent in the fabric of the patient's life, leaving the patient stunned and adrift. There
is thus often a clear collapse in the patient's functioning and general life trajectory
surrounding the death of the other. It may have begun with the patient leaving a
career path to care for a dying and not necessarily cooperative or grateful relative; the death of a tyrannical, critical parent; or some other conflictual situation,
such as the death of a child for which the patient, fairly or not, blames himself or
herself.

Perhaps because of having studiously avoided thoughts and feelings about the
death, the image of the deceased that the patient presents often tends to be cursory and even cartoonish: "She was an angel" or "She was a witch." The task of the
therapist is to help the patient develop a more three-dimensional, more nuanced,
and more emotionally meaningful portrait of the dead person and the relationship they had.

Questions to ask include: How did the patient handle the mourning process? What are the patient's feelings about the deceased: is there a range of emotions, including some negative affect? Does the patient feel he or she has grieved, or respond by saying, "Well, I was too busy with this pandemic . . ."?

Treatment

If you and the patient choose complicated bereavement as a focus, the goals of treatment are twofold:

(1) Catharsis: to help the patient experience his or her feelings of loss; and
(2) To find a new, "post mortem" path forward, including new relationships or activities to replace the lost one.

In essence, catharsis is giving the patient space and encouragement to reflect on and tolerate powerful feelings about the death and the dead person. It can begin with an exploration of how the person died. Because patients with complicated grief generally suffer from extreme guilt, it is important to explore what the patient's role was in the time leading up to, during, and following the death. *Where was the patient when he or she learned of the death?* Patients frequently feel they should have done something, or shouldn't have done something, and that now it's too late to change.

Ask the patient who the deceased person was, and how the patient felt about the deceased. It's easier to start with positive feelings: Why might the patient miss the person? What was good about their relationship? Prime the pump of the patient's emotional memories and allow the patient to reflect. On occasion this suffices to get the patient going. Often patients with complicated bereavement avoid negative affects, feeling the emotions themselves are bad and reflect badly on themselves: "What a terrible person I am to be angry at a dead person who can no longer defend herself!" After having focused on the positive, you can reassure the patient that relationships are complex, people have a range of feelings about each other, and it's okay, even important to talk about them.

"Even the best of relationships has difficulties; no two people get along all the time. Tell me about some of the friction you and he may have had."

Successfully tapping into pent up emotions often unleashes them in a flood that can panic not only patients but therapists. Yet this onrush represents the potential success of treatment. The goal of the therapist, once having opened the floodgates, is to sit tight and maintain poise. Demonstrate that *feelings are powerful but not dangerous* by listening sympathetically and silently, perhaps with brow furrowed or tears in your eyes. Say nothing and do nothing to interrupt this outflow. To hurriedly offer the patient a box of tissues (which remote therapy thankfully prevents) or to interrupt the patient with a question or comment that changes the topic ("How old was your mother?") demonstrates the kind of affect avoidance you are working to prevent, and works against the treatment by suggesting that the emotions you are eliciting are too frightening for you to tolerate. If you can hang in there, looking concerned, caring, and unfrightened (implying "I've seen this before, and it's distressing but not dangerous"), you and the patient will end the session feeling emotionally drained, but that you've been through something important together. The interrupted or avoided mourning process restarts in a session like this. You will have provided immense social support, and the patient is likely to feel exhausted but decompressed, relieved. Subsequent sessions may repeat this process, but it's generally a lot easier, the pressure relieved.

You can encourage the patient (without assigning homework) to do things that remind them of the deceased and their relationship and hence evoke feelings: looking at photographs, visiting meaningful places where they had spent time, perhaps going to (virtual) church if that's helpful. As the patient talks about feelings, symptoms are likely to decrease. The deceased comes into more realistic focus. The patient feels sad, perhaps angry, hurt, or disappointed, but no longer depressed in the same way. Serial measurement of symptoms can confirm this.

Now the task shifts, at least in part, to the question, *Where does the patient want to go from here?* You can't replace a lost parent or child, whose absence creates a gap in the patient's life. What the patient can do is find new relationships or activities that to some degree fill that gap: not a substitution, but a new gratification, support, or interest. What does the patient want to do with the time previously spent with the deceased? Sometimes mourners decide to volunteer for a medical charity like the American Cancer Society to honor the deceased. (It's not yet clear what the Covid-19 equivalent of this will be.) The challenge during the pandemic is that it's harder to start new relationships or new activities during a lockdown, but the patient can nonetheless make plans and begin to implement them. You can still meet people online. For patients who have suffered the death of a significant other due to Covid-19, there are innumerable constructive ways to join the rebuilding process that society will require in its aftermath.

ROLE DISPUTE

As discussed in Chapter 3, role disputes occur when there is an imbalance in an important relationship, with the patient invariably on the losing end. Whether this is a trigger or a consequence of symptoms does not matter: in IPT, we are always interested in the connection between the two, not in etiology per se. Because depression and anxiety impair self-assertion and raise fears of abandonment, patients with mood and anxiety disorders have difficulty in expressing their needs and their disinclinations. That leaves relationships in a disequilibrium where other people's needs get met, not the patient's.

The patient often resents this situation but feels that there's nothing to be done. Self-assertion feels "selfish," which is bad: even having the wish for selfish things reveals a character flaw in the patient's eyes. Asking for something is likely only to lead to rejection and could perhaps ruin or even end the relationship. The patient also typically lacks comfort in negotiating such needs. Thus a relationship that could potentially provide social support becomes instead its opposite, a problem that contributes to and perpetuates symptoms. As with the other IPT problem areas, a strong psychosocial literature establishes the connection between troubled relationships and depressive and other psychiatric symptoms.[69]

History

In collecting the interpersonal inventory, explore how the patient gets along with others, both at better moments and particularly in the current episode. How comfortable is he or she in saying, "I'd like" or "I don't like" anything? How does he or she handle disagreements? Many patients will concede: "I don't do confrontation"; "I really don't do anger." The proud statement, "We've never had a fight" is a warning flag.

If a relationship with a partner, a family member, a boss or work colleague, or a friend appears conflicted, problematic, and important to the narrative of the current psychiatric episode, *role dispute* may provide a helpful treatment format.

Get a sense of what has been good and bad in the relationship. How did the two meet? How intimate are they with one another? (Do they confide at all?) How, in the patient's view, do they get along? What relationship patterns exist, particularly surrounding points of disagreement? Many confrontation-aversive depressed and anxious patients feel they have only two options: either to accept an uncomfortable relationship, or to leave. Diagnose the stage of the dispute: some dysfunctional relationships are overtly problematic; others covertly so. The two opponents may be in open conflict (*renegotiation* stage); or in a kind of cold war stalemate (*impasse*), distant and barely speaking; or breaking up (*dissolution*).[7] How you approach the dispute will depend upon what's going on.

Treatment

Explore the relationship. What is going wrong? What does the patient want to happen? (What's a realistic goal?) The opening question ("How have things been since we last met?") of each session, like the rounds in a boxing match, will often yield an update on the latest chapter in the ongoing dispute and how the patient is feeling about it. Elicit and normalize those feelings: the patient's difficulty in tolerating negative affects is often part of the difficulty and can be blamed on the mood or anxiety disorder or PTSD. If the patient feels hurt, disappointed, resentful, is that a reasonable and warranted response to the events? If so, what can he or she *do* with that feeling? (What options exist?) Role play is crucial to prepare a patient to express these feelings, which often have been expressed only partly, ineffectually (e.g., with sarcasm or sullen withdrawal), or not at all, rather than in an assertive statement of how the patient feels and what the patient would like.

Psychoeducation should be employed judiciously, in small bits, but it can be helpful—*after* the patient has described anger, or disappointment, or hurt feelings—to explain the concept of a role dispute. What follows is too much psychoeducation for a single session but could be apportioned across several sessions:

Relationships. "Relationships are complicated, because even generally compatible people differ in their desires and dislikes. Good relationships are based on healthy compromise: no one gets everything they want, but both parties can achieve sufficient satisfaction and feel they're a team. *This requires good communication of feelings.* Depression [or anxiety, or PTSD] can make it hard to ask for what you need, or to express your dislikes of the other person's behavior. Conversely, too imbalanced a relationship may bring out these symptoms [which would involve abusive behavior in PTSD]."

Desires. "It's okay to want things; *a certain degree of "selfishness" is healthy and protective.* No one likes people who are selfish all the time, but you're in no danger of that: your danger lies in asking for too little. Being too self*less* leaves you in danger of being a martyr. *If you don't say what you want, you're much less likely to have your needs met.*"

Anger. "If someone does something that bothers you and you don't tell the person, you end up holding in that festering annoyance. That doesn't help your mood. Worse, because the person hasn't gotten your feedback, he or she will very likely repeat the bothersome behavior, and can be excused for doing so because people *expect* to hear when someone doesn't like what they're doing. So if you have reason to feel annoyed and you tell the person, you accomplish several things: you get the feeling off your chest, which feels good; you set a boundary with the other person, who then stands informed that you don't like what he or she is doing, and may change the behavior and stop bothering you. If they don't, it makes it even more reasonable for you to get angry when they do it again.

"If you feel you've been mistreated, you can tell the other person and ask for an apology. That may help determine how understanding and trustworthy that person is."

Patients generally recognize that expressing one's feelings is, at least in theory, a reasonable approach. The trick is to introduce these concepts as the patient recounts the emotional experience, so that it's more than just an intellectual concept.

If the patient and the other person are at an impasse, mutually withdrawn, it may be necessary to increase conflict in the relationship acutely in order to try to change it. This is worth explaining and predicting to the patient. Encouraging the patient to try to communicate with the other may stir up strife, but it clarifies what the issues are and how the patient can approach them.

With adequate role play, including exploration of contingencies, the patient is likely to be able to renegotiate the relationship to his or her greater satisfaction. Should this fail, the patient will at least recognize that it's not for lack of a good faith effort on his or her own part, and that the problem may lie with the other person—relieving self-blame. If the relationship remains truly unsatisfactory despite their best efforts, some patients will decide to end the relationship (dissolution) and find an alternative. Sometimes leaving a job or a marriage, however difficult a transition, is the best thing to do. If the patient decides to end the relationship, that itself is an important emotional negotiation, which exploring options and role play may help, and the termination shifts to a role transition in which the patient mourns what has been lost and appreciates the potential for new gains.

The setting of disaster alters relationships and provides new opportunities for role disputes of various kinds. Some patients have reported an easing of tensions with difficult bosses or coworkers during the pandemic because work has slowed and they are no longer occupying the same physical space. On the other hand, many find that existing problems at home are magnified by constant proximity to family members, by added tasks of homeschooling, housework, and the like. As noted in Chapter 2, it may be hard for patients to find privacy to discuss difficult marriages when their partner is in the next room. Several of my patients had been involved in budding romances that have been strained, put on hold, or possibly have ended because of Covid-19. In some cases, one member of the relationship moved out of the city to escape the virus; in others, formerly trivial geographic distance has become a major obstacle with fears about using public transport. Friendships have been strained by lack of available joint activities as the city has shut down. People complain that there's really nothing to talk about: all there is the virus.

ROLE TRANSITION

A role transition is a broad category, including any significant life change that alters the individual's sense of life trajectory. This could mean beginning or ending a job or relationship, getting married or divorced, developing a medical illness, moving to a new geographic setting, etc. Clearly the advent of a plague and its extended social consequences constitute a role transition, which may entail any or many of the job, relationship, health, and other changes just listed. Thus any patient presenting in the context of this disaster is likely to fit the category of role transition, although it may feel more clinically appropriate to use the complicated bereavement or role dispute formats in particular cases.

Treating a role transition is akin to treating complicated bereavement, except that no one has died. In both instances, it's important for the patient to mourn what has been lost (the old social role) and to try to appreciate the benefits of the new role. This can appear difficult, as the depressed or traumatized patient invariably sees the past as halcyon and the present as awful. Yet change is complex, and there are trade-offs to every change. Even objectively bad events—like the coronavirus pandemic—can turn out to have silver linings. We were impressed in our 1998 treatment study of depression during the height of the AIDS epidemic that depressed HIV-positive patients with minimal T-cell counts, no available effective antiviral treatment, and the possibility of an early death from a highly stigmatized infection, who had seen friends and lovers die of the same infection they now had, who had fevers, Kaposi's sarcoma, encroaching visual loss, and recurrent superinfections, were nonetheless able to find meaning in the midst of that viral epidemic and to take steps to improve their lives and mood.[68] They liked the "can do" approach of IPT and, perhaps because of the extreme pressure under which they found themselves, they were willing to take bold steps ("live dangerously") in IPT. They developed new and better relationships (in some cases for the first time), mourned and established memorials for partners and friends, and made the most of whatever time they might have left.

History

The presence of a role transition should be easy to establish under disastrous circumstances. A group of concomitant role transitions seems more likely: occupational change plus social change plus illness in the family, for example. If so, all can be grouped under the same rubric, as we did with depressed HIV-positive patients.

> "All hell has broken loose, and your life has turned upside down. We call that a role transition."

Treatment

As noted in Chapter 3, patients in a role transition feel out of control, overwhelmed by change that they experience as chaos. Simply reframing this chaos as a role transition—a period of change to which the individual can react and adapt—can be a therapeutic maneuver. Things were one way, now they're another, and the change is indeed upsetting, but as you adjust to this transition things should calm down. Again, adjusting means recognizing what has been lost (the old role of having a job, feeling important in the office; or of having been in a relationship that's now over, etc.) and mourning the fact of the transition itself ("Why did this have to happen, now, to my life?!"). Give the patient room to express these feelings. Don't rush in with virtual tissues; feelings are powerful, but not dangerous. Let the patient experience them and learn that for himself or herself.

Adjusting to a role transition also means trying to figure out how best to handle the new role: not working, working from home while trying to take care of children whose school has closed, caring for a partner with Covid-19 infection or struggling to recover from it oneself are examples that come to mind. These are stressful and challenging situations likely to evoke strong feelings. Encourage the patient to tolerate and express those feelings ("Of course upsetting circumstances like X upset you. Tell me how you're feeling about that. . . . What kind of 'upset'?"). Does the patient have confidants or allies who can provide social support in getting through this difficult moment? Further, what does the patient want to do under these circumstances that might improve the situation? Are there ways to enlist help from others? To make beneficial life changes, including new relationships and new, wished-for directions?

Depressed, anxious, and traumatized individuals tend to undervalue their capabilities and surprise themselves with their accomplishments in just a few weeks of IPT. They often emerge from role transitions feeling they have achieved changes they never thought possible in the midst of chaos and chaotic symptoms. They may come away with a new view of themselves as survivors, veterans, as tougher and more capable than they had previously thought they were.

Note that, regardless of problem area, the basic IPT strategies are the same:

- Organize the treatment around a life crisis (interpersonal focus);
- Elicit the patient's feelings, let the patient sit with them, and normalize them as responses to particular interpersonal encounters; and
- Then help the patient plan to act on them, resolving the crisis.

It's a matter of learning to trust your feelings—as these patients invariably do not—and to use them to handle life.

In the next chapters (5–7) we will apply these problem areas to the treatment of patients with differing diagnoses presenting in the context of the pandemic. I present these in the order of their supporting IPT evidence: patients with major depression, PTSD, and anxiety disorders. As these disorders often are comorbid with one another, which IPT variant you choose to approach the patient with may depend upon which disorder or life circumstances appear most salient. Because the general approach is the same, treating one part of the picture tends to generally relieve symptomatology.[e.g.,10]

5

Major Depression

Depression is where IPT began. Major depressive disorder consists not only of neurovegetative and cognitive but of affective and interpersonal symptoms. Depressed patients feel uncomfortable with other people, afraid their depression will show and reveal them to be "bad." It takes a tremendous effort—at a time when energy and initiative are lacking—to act normal and pleasant under such circumstances. Even when such behavior succeeds, the patient often feels fraudulent for having "faked" an encounter; if he or she knew how the patient really felt, who the patient really was, the other person would reject the patient utterly.[102] Meanwhile, the general depressive tendency is to withdraw from people altogether, diminishing needed social support.

Stressors related to the pandemic, or combined with those of the pandemic, can take their toll. As the previous chapters have already described the basic IPT techniques for treating major depression, their use is best illustrated here with case examples.

COMPLICATED BEREAVEMENT

Ms. A, a fifty-nine-year-old widowed Methodist African-American New York City transit worker and mother of one, presented in May 2020 (on Zoom) with the chief complaint: "It's been hard since my mother died." Her eighty-two-year-old mother, who had lived with her for the past nine years, had fallen ill with what proved to be Covid-19 infection in March 2020. Ms. A had taken off days from work and had done her best to nurse her until her mother needed hospitalization for respiratory distress and high fevers. On the third day of the hospitalization, the hospital banned family visits. Because her mother required intubation and a respirator, they could not speak by phone. A week later, Ms. A learned that her mother had died in the hospital—alone.

They were regular churchgoers, but the pandemic had shuttered her church. Most of her family lived in the South and could not travel to New York during the pandemic. Her minister arranged a Skype funeral, but Ms. A found it forced and did not cry or feel as comforted as she had expected. Her friends and some coworkers called her, dropped off food, but were reluctant to visit a house that had been infected during the lockdown. Ms. A herself developed a slight cough, but a nasal swab test was negative for Covid-19.

She felt horrible, worrying that she had brought the virus home from her transit route and had caused her mother's death. She felt that she had failed her mother, having been unable to see her in her final days, and felt cut off from her usually supportive community. She reported a depressed and anxious mood, low energy, poor appetite and concentration, and had withdrawn to her bed, where she spent most of the day feeling "half dead." Spiritually opposed to suicide, she nonetheless felt her life was empty, would have been happy to "pass in my sleep," and had thoughts of reunion with her mother in the afterlife. Her Ham-D Scale score was 27, in the severe range.

Her therapist said, "What a terrible loss, under such terrible circumstances! No wonder you're so upset! . . . Please tell me about you and your mother." Ms. A felt that it was too fresh and painful to really talk about, that her heart was breaking. The therapist waited, looking sad. After a while, Ms. A began to describe what it was like growing up in the Carolinas with her Mama, a single parent of four, how she went hungry at times to feed the children, and how sad and brave her mother had been when her younger brother died of pneumonia when Ms. A was seven. Most of the memories, though, were happy. "My Mama was strict, but she was good, and had the biggest heart in the world."

Her history revealed that Ms. A had been depressed once before, in her twenties following a miscarriage (another interpersonal loss), but had recovered with family and church support and without formal treatment. She had siblings and other relatives down South, a thirty-two-year-old married daughter and an eight-year-old grandchild living in another borough of New York City, and numerous friends in her neighborhood and church. Her tendency, though, was to keep her feelings to herself rather than risk burdening others. There was a family history of mood and some substance disorder, although Ms. A rarely drank alcohol and used no other drugs. She had mild, controlled hypertension, was slightly overweight, but was generally in good physical condition, without a thyroid history.

On mental status, Ms. A appeared on the screen alert, well groomed, and simply but neatly dressed in black. Her movements were somewhat agitated, her speech fluent and unpressured, and she largely avoided eye contact. Her mood was depressed and anxious with a reactive, often tearful, nonlabile affect that she struggled to contain. Her thinking was goal directed but characterized by hopelessness, with passive suicidal ideation but no plan or intent. Her sensorium was clear, her intelligence greater than average.

At the end of the first session of history taking, the therapist summarized:

"Losing your mother is a terrible thing, and having it happen in the midst of this pandemic really doesn't help. You're cut off from a lot of your supports, which is a problem, and staying home has disrupted your daily routine, which is a problem. I know you don't feel like reaching out when you're feeling so depressed, but social support is a real need at a time like this. It's hard enough to go through such a loss without having to do it alone. And if you can get on a little more of a regular schedule, give yourself some structure, that would probably help you feel better too."

At the end of the second session, after further reviewing her story, patient and therapist agreed that Ms. A had suffered multiple losses, but that her mother's death was the hardest:

"You've told me a lot; please tell me if I'm getting the big picture. You're a strong individual, and you've gotten through a lot of losses in your life - - your father's leaving when you were little, your brother's death, the mis- carriage, your husband's death – but this is the worst. You were so close to your mother, and you feel responsible for her death. And at a time when it would have been really important to have support from your family and community, the pandemic has cut you off. So you've been overwhelmed by this grief—this is what we call complicated bereave- ment, a type of depression. It's not your fault, and you have an excellent chance of getting better with treatment. I suggest that we spend the re- maining ten sessions doing Interpersonal Psychotherapy, a brief treat- ment that focuses on grief, working on how you can come to terms with this terrible event, particularly under such difficult circumstances.

"As part of treatment, I'm going to encourage you to pay attention to your feelings, even the painful ones, because they tell you something impor- tant about what's going on. If you lose someone close to you, it's got to hurt, and part of getting through this period is accepting that emotion. The more you deal with your feelings, the less painful they're like to get. So I encourage you to think of memories, maybe look at photographs or other things that remind you of your mother, and we can talk about the feelings they raise."

Ms. A. agreed.

On the Covid Checklist (Box 3.2 in Chapter 3), she was worried about Covid-19 infection given her relatively high-risk job, but had taken time off from work. Her sleep cycle had been disturbed by the mood disorder, with difficulty falling asleep and staying asleep, and by her spending much of the day in bed. She did, guiltily, feel she should return to work. Her church and other social contacts had been cut off by the lockdown. She was not active on social media.

Middle Phase

The early sessions of the middle phase focused on the strengths of Ms. A's bond with her mother. She was the youngest of four children and only daughter, the favored "baby" of the family. That also meant spending more time with her mother doing household work while her brothers studied or played. Her mother confided in her and made her feel loved. She also insisted she needed to get an education, to avoid drugs and street violence. When Ms. A and her husband decided to move to New York, she and her mother had a tearful goodbye and stayed regularly in touch, first by phone, and eventually by FaceTime. Her mother regularly sent her greeting cards expressing her love. "My Mama was my rock." When Ms. A's husband died, her mother moved to New York to be with her and help with childcare, and continued to live with her even after her granddaughter grew up and left the home. Her mother's presence had helped Ms. A cope with the death of her husband: she was able to grieve without becoming depressed.

The therapist asked in more detail about the events leading up to her mother's death, and Ms. A's reaction to them. She burst into tears. "I feel so guilty—we knew she could get the virus, being old, and I told her I'd stay home from work, but she said I needed to work and she'd be okay. I'm sure I gave her the virus. I'm sure I killed her. My own mother!" She recounted trying to care for her ailing mother at home and her mother's lack of cooperation as she became more panicky about breathing, calling for the ambulance and taking her to the hospital, and being cut off from her mother at the ER door. She visited her in the hospital—which was hard to reach during the lockdown—for the first two days, but on the third was barred entry by hospital policy, an attempt to limit the spread of Covid-19. Thereafter she was frantic, frequently calling the hospital nursing station on an overwhelmed unit where staff rarely answered the phone. Then the numb feeling of learning her mother had died. The therapist listened silently and sympathetically, feeling quite sad but resisting the urge to interrupt with something comforting, letting Ms. A weep and recount her memories. It was painful and draining, but Ms. A seemed somewhat relieved by the end of the session.

In response to "How have things been since we last met?" at the start of the next session, Ms. A reported still feeling sad and guilty, but feeling "a little less heavy" after the previous session. She had begun to return to work, was on a more regular sleep and work schedule, but was not talking about her feelings with her coworkers. The therapist asked: "Can you tell me about the guilt you're feeling? . . . What do you feel you should have or shouldn't have done?" Ms. A tearfully blamed herself for her mother's infection and terrible death. One reason she had not talked more with her family and friends is that she felt sure they would blame her as well. The therapist did not interrupt or contradict her but explored the details of the situation. Late in the session, Ms. A paused and herself raised the contradiction: if she had infected her mother, then why had her own Covid-19 test been negative? The therapist nodded and looked curious: "That's an interesting point. What about that?" At the end of the session, he added: "I understand your concern that you might have inadvertently infected your mother, and it is hard to know with an invisible virus. But you raised a really good point: How could you have infected her if you're not infected yourself? And I do want to remind you that guilt is a symptom of depression, question 2 on the Hamilton Depression Rating Scale."

The patient said, "I hear you, but I still feel guilty. I would never want to hurt my Mama." But she looked somewhat relieved.

In subsequent sessions Ms. A appeared less, if still, depressed. She was now working full time, which felt both anxiety-provoking because of the viral threat and comforting that she was continuing to help the community. She liked the human contact of her job. Ms. A placed a family portrait, a photograph of her mother, herself, and her teenage daughter in cap and gown, in front of her computer screen for the therapist to see. "This was at Halle's high school graduation," she said. "We all had a great day, and it made me and Mama so proud. She made a big meal and baked her special coconut cake." Ms. A burst into tears, but she also smiled. She looked less physically tense.

They began to discuss whether she could share some of these memories with family members or friends. Ms. A was hesitant on two grounds: her general wish to be strong and not burden people and her subsiding but still guilty sense that she was to blame. She agreed, though, that the funeral hadn't been sufficient relief and that it was hard to carry around such strong feelings on her own. It hadn't been like that when her brother or her husband died. Her daughter had actually tried to talk to her about her grandmother's death, but Ms. A had changed the subject.

They role played how this might go with her daughter, who was living in another borough, hard to reach under current circumstances. "How much have you talked with Halle about what happened and how you've felt?" asked the therapist. "What might you like to say to her?" Ms. A responded, "I guess I'd start telling her what Mama meant, means, to me. And that I feel to blame for what happened. . . ." After she had finished, the therapist asked: "How did that sound to you? . . . Did you say what you wanted to say? Anything you'd add or leave out? . . . What did you think about your tone, the way you said it?"

She did talk to her daughter, who didn't blame her for Mama's death, and both of them agreed they felt better for it. By session 6, Ms. A's Ham-D score had dropped to 16, a considerable improvement if still in the moderately symptomatic range. Noting that she was not fully out of the woods yet, the therapist congratulated Ms. A on her progress. "You're getting better, and no wonder, with the way you're handling things. Keep it up!"

They began to discuss not only what she loved about her mother but some irritations, which Ms. A was initially reluctant to raise. "We don't say bad things about those who've passed." The therapist encouraged her that no relationship was perfect, that people who really loved each other could still get on each other's nerves at times. Ms. A thought for a while. She said could be annoyed at her mother for favoring her daughter over her at times. She didn't like that her mother smoked in the apartment—and denied it, despite the lingering tobacco smell. She had felt guilty for feeling angry toward her mother when she fell ill with Covid-19 and wouldn't cooperate with treatment. (The therapist noted that her mother might have been delirious, but that it must have been frustrating nonetheless.) Ms. A also reported talking to family and friends more, and confiding in some of them.

Termination

By the end of treatment, her Ham-D score had fallen to 5, in the normal range. Ms. A was still sad about her mother, missed her terribly, but now understood this as mourning—and no longer felt guilty or depressed. She understood, too, that this mourning would continue for the rest of her life, and that strong feelings and memories might come back in waves and on anniversaries, but that her grief was already transforming now that she was dealing with it. Her memories of her mother were one way of keeping her spirit alive. Life felt worth living despite the loss and despite the strictures of the pandemic. She had fully resumed work, was attending virtual church services, and arranged to walk with her daughter and granddaughter at arm's length. She was involved again in her social circle. She felt more comfortable both in tolerating her own feelings and in expressing them to others: "Being strong doesn't mean I can't tell people how I feel; in fact, maybe that *is* being strong."

ROLE DISPUTE

Ms. B, a 46-year-old white Protestant advertising executive who commuted to work in New York from Connecticut, presented with recurrent major depression (Ham-D= 28) and chief complaint: "I'm sorry. . . I'm trying to be a good sport."

Ms. B had been married for nearly twenty years to George, a businessman who had had a debilitating stroke four years earlier that left him partially incapacitated and essentially housebound. She had taken leave from work to care for him, but then struggled to have him accept home health aides so that she could return to work. He was in great denial about the extent of his illness, saying he didn't need assistance, yet constantly entreating Ms. B for help. She had a long history of caretaking, beginning with her own father's illness in her childhood, had been depressed in the past, and tended to put the needs of others before her own. Ms. B's own mother had been a very angry woman, screaming and breaking things over sometimes minor frustrations, and Ms. B had vowed never to act that way herself. After some months of caring for her post-stroke husband with the help (and burden) of three teenage children and a part-time health aide, while struggling to maintain her career, she had developed major depression. She eventually saw her general practitioner for a check-up, who gave her fluoxetine 10 mg and encouraged her to return to work. Both interventions had helped.

Their warm but always fractious marriage had shown the strain, but for several years she had occupied herself with her career and raising her children. There were still happy moments in the marriage despite George's cognitive and physical limitations. The two truly loved each other. Then, when the coronavirus hit and she was forced to "shelter in place" at home, she found herself in constant contact with her increasingly irritable, demanding, and gradually declining husband. The kids were home all the time for remote schooling, and tempers frayed. "My house is like a pressure cooker, and the longer it goes on, the worse it gets."

Her work had suffered from her disrupted sleep and concentration, but she managed to function. She felt overly criticized by the head of her firm but felt this was something she had to live with. She had friends, some of them real confidants, but had been cut off from them by the pandemic. Her husband's medical frailty made her particularly cautious about physical isolation to avoid infection. "There's nothing to do, nothing to talk about except the virus—we're all sick of that." She and her friends did not feel comfortable meeting for masked walks, and she was no longer commuting in to work. The therapist asked how she fought with people when they disagreed. "Oh, I don't fight. I don't do confrontation."

The therapist looked puzzled. "So, when you disagree . . .?"

MS. B: "I try to walk away. Sometimes I exercise, that helps. But you really only have two choices: either you put up with it or you leave."

THERAPIST: "Then it must *really* be a pressure cooker at home. How do you feel when George asks you to do something for him from the next room, even with the aide or your kids right next to him?"

MS. B: "It bothers me. But that's the way he is. You have to accept people and not ask them to do more than they can. You can't change people."

THERAPIST: "Really? . . . But how does it feel?"

MS. B: "I feel annoyed, but that's not a helpful feeling. It's not productive to feel that way. Besides, it's not his fault he had a stroke, I can't blame him for that."

The therapist paused and let that sink in. Then he said:

"No wonder you're feeling depressed. You're trapped in the house during a pandemic, you love your husband but he bothers you and there's no way for you to push back. You're trying to be a 'good sport,' but how long can you keep it up under these circumstances?"

MS. B: "It's getting really hard."

THERAPIST: "There's probably a way for you to improve the situation, which is likely to improve your mood, too. That sounds like a problem to work on."

MS. B: "That would be a relief. But I don't see any way to do it, it just looks hopeless."

Ms. B appeared her stated age. She was alert, well-groomed in a business suit on the screen, with appropriate make-up that began to streak when she cried. Her movements were tense and agitated, her speech clipped and controlled, with pauses during which she said she was distracted by negative thoughts about the hopelessness of her life. Her mood was depressed and anxious, with a somewhat constricted affect that gave way to short floods of tears. In describing tension with her husband she displayed no hint of anger. Her thinking was grossly goal-directed but distractible, clearly pessimistic, often hopeless in its tenor. She tended to shy away from painful feelings, but acknowledged they were there. Ms. B acknowledged passive suicidal ideation "but I'd never do it to my family." Her sensorium was grossly clear.

The therapist increased Ms. B's fluoxetine dosage from 10 to 20 mg every morning, which she tolerated without side effects. They also tried adding trazodone 50 mg for sleep, which she found intolerable. After the second session, in which they reviewed further history, the therapist offered Ms. B a formulation. He had recognized that she was clearly experiencing a role transition during the pandemic (as everyone was), but one of its most deleterious effects had been to heighten the acrimony in her increasingly one-sided relationship with her husband. This was what she seemed to find most distressing. He therefore framed the problem to her as a role dispute:

"Thank you for telling me so much about your life; please tell me if I'm understanding you. You have had a good but difficult marriage, difficult particularly since George had the stroke four years ago—that's when you first got depressed. It's hard for you to disagree with people, you want to help them, and it seems really hard to disagree with a husband who's had such medical problems. But it's been hard living with that at times, and particularly in the last couple of months when you've been locked in the house with him and your independent routine has suffered from the pandemic. The Covid disaster has affected you in a variety of ways, but the worst is that it's made your marriage more difficult to tolerate. Is that fair?"

MS. B: "Yes, that's right. That's fair."

THERAPIST: "We call the struggle you're in with George a *role dispute.*
A good relationship should involve compromise by both parties, so that both get their needs met. What seems to have happened in your marriage is that your husband is getting his needs met, at some unfair cost to you. It's hard for you to tell him how you'd like things to be, and hard for you to say no to him. No wonder you're suffering if you're feeling trapped, resentful, but see no way out. What you can do, over our remaining twelve weekly sessions, is to figure out how to renegotiate the relationship so that it works to both of your advantages and better fulfills both of your needs. It may mean doing some things that will make you uncomfortable, but in the end that may turn out to be good. It would mean paying attention to feelings of resentment and anger, since those aren't feelings that come up at random: that tells you when you're feeling mistreated, or things are unfair. If you can recognize that anger and turn it to use, the marriage may go better and you may feel better. Does that make sense to you?"

MS. B: "It sort of makes sense. You're right that I don't like being angry. I don't think I can do it, but I guess I can try."

Beyond defining the time frame and focus of IPT, the therapist also reviewed the Covid Checklist (Box 3.2 in Chapter 3).

1. Ms. B was at relatively low risk for getting coronavirus infection during the lockdown, but she worried about leaving the house at all lest she inadvertently put her medically compromised husband at risk. Yet staying home increased their friction, robbing her of the long walks she used to take to blow off steam and relieve muscle tension. She took appropriate precautions when she did go out, wearing a mask and gloves, and showering when she returned home. Patient and therapist agreed that there was room for some anxiety, but that perhaps she could take socially distanced walks for her own health. Her needs had to count too.

2. The lockdown had considerably affected Ms. B's daily routine. It had cost her the social architecture of commuting, which she had once regretted took more than an hour each way but now realized had been in some ways relaxing, allowing her to unwind after a busy day and giving her some space from George. Lack of exercise and depressive symptoms had disrupted her sleep cycle. They discussed sleep hygiene and regularizing her schedule as being likely to help her mood.

3. The pandemic had unquestionably affected her social bonds. Particularly since her husband's infirmity, she had been dependent on social relationships. On the one hand, she no longer saw work colleagues and friends, who provided companionship and varying degrees of social support. Communication had become more difficult not just because of physical separation, but because she didn't want to burden friends with her "misery" and was embarrassed to talk about how bad things felt at home. The head of the firm had developed a mass Zoom meeting approach to conducting business that made it hard to speak to him more personally. On the other hand, she was if anything seeing too much of her family, exacerbating her role dispute with her husband. She was getting along pretty well with her children, "even though they're in their teens."

4. Having become regularly discouraged whenever she tuned in to the medical and political news, Ms. B had decided to restrict herself to the *New York Times* each morning. Thus she was not suffering from excessive media exposure.

Middle Phase

Treatment thereafter focused on the marriage. "How have you been since we last met?" elicited George's sometimes carping and petulant demands, to which she responded with resigned compliance. Each time, the therapist pushed for Ms. B's feelings, and she increasingly recognized her resentment. "It's one-sided, but what can I do about it? He's pretty helpless." They discussed this. George had a hemi-plegic limp but could in fact walk around the house and manage many things him-self, yet he seemed to wait until she was involved in her remote business work to interrupt with minor requests. Ms. B's career was precious to her, and she worried that she was "starting to get old for my industry" and might get shunted aside or even lose her job if she didn't devote herself to it. This was a particular concern now that she was the family breadwinner and the pandemic had upset their finances.

THERAPIST: "Are those reasonable concerns?"

MS. B: "I think so. I have to carry the responsibility."

THERAPIST: "And when George interrupts your work to ask you to get him a snack?"

MS. B: "I get annoyed. But, you know, I don't like getting angry, I feel bad arguing with a sick man, and I'm worried that if I really push back I'll puncture his denial and he'll get really depressed."

THERAPIST: "Depressed the way you've gotten depressed? With a Hamilton score of 28?"

MS. B: "Well, no, maybe not that bad. But I don't want to upset him."

THERAPIST: "Should you *not* feel annoyed if you're trying to do your job, which is hard enough when you're feeling this way—and he then bothers you for something he could actually handle himself?"

MS. B: "No, it's reasonable. I know it's reasonable. I just don't like the feeling."

THERAPIST: [after waiting for thirty seconds, observing] "It's an uncomfort-able feeling, but it tells you what's going on."

MS. B: "It isn't really fair, what he's doing."

THERAPIST: "I agree with you. . . . So what options do you have at a moment like that?"

MS. B: "I try to ignore it. Or I take a break from work and get him what he wants. But then I'm actually angrier."

THERAPIST: [after another pause] "Good point. Does that make sense, that you might be angrier?"

MS. B: "Yes, it's like he's won and I'm his servant."

THERAPIST: "So that doesn't feel good. Are there other options? What else might you try?"

MS. B: "Sometimes I'd like to say: 'Look, I'm in the middle of something im-portant. Ask someone else to do it. Or do it yourself!' But then I'd feel terrible."

THERAPIST: "Why?"

MS. B: "We keep getting back to this. He's had a stroke, I don't like to fight . . . "

Note how, as often happens, a role play emerged from the basic IPT paradigm of linking and exploring feelings and life events. The therapist then followed this up:

"How did what you just said sound to you? . . . Are those the words you'd like to use? . . . What about your tone of voice? . . . And suppose George answered by saying, 'I can't do that,' '. . . but I really need your help,' or . . . 'You don't care about me at all'?"

They repeated the role play a couple of times, after which Ms. B said she felt more comfortable. The therapist suggested that anger was a signal necessary to self-defense: if she couldn't express it, she was at the mercy of other people's needs. Expressing anger/annoyance/frustration didn't necessarily mean screaming at anyone, and she certainly wasn't screaming in the role plays. It just meant stating her needs, what she wanted and didn't want. It was self-defense. Ms. B agreed, at least in theory, but looked wary.

It also emerged that Ms. B felt guilty at getting angry at a sick man. "It isn't his fault he had a stroke—although of course he was a smoker. . . . But I don't want to blame him for what he really can't do." The therapist complimented her on her compassion, then asked whether George's illness gave him carte blanche to behave any way he'd like. And even if the debility wasn't George's fault, did that mean she wasn't going to feel annoyed by his distractions? Ms. B thought hard about this. "I want to be forgiving and understanding, but it shouldn't mean I have to be a martyr," she decided. Maybe it was okay to get angry at him, even if he had medical debility?

Ms. B came in the following week and talked about work issues. She came up with a tentative plan for speaking one on one with the head of the firm and role played that.

In the following session, Ms. B returned on Zoom in a somewhat less depressed and calmer mood. George had asked her to make him a sandwich in the midst of an important conference call. She had waved him off, and afterward tried to confront him, asking him not to interrupt her work. He had basically ignored her: "But I need you to do this for me! I'm really hungry." Flustered, she had given in and made the sandwich. This left her both more discouraged and angrier. When, an hour later, George again interrupted a work call, asking that she make him tea, she felt "so frustrated that, without stopping to think, I gave him one of the speeches we've been practicing. I'm not sure it was perfect, but it had an effect."

Ms. B reported having said something along the lines of: "George, can't you see I'm in the middle of my work? I told you, I need to do this right now. If you need help, please ask one of the kids to help you. And look, when you interrupt me like this, it makes me angry, it feels disrespectful. I need to go back to my work right now, but let's talk about this later, okay?"

George backed off, and she felt relieved. She had not in fact carried the discussion with George further, but he had not interrupted her work in the following two days.

THERAPIST: "So how are you feeling about this?"
MS. B: "Good! Though it feels like a fragile truce. But I was glad I said something. I didn't get too angry, and nothing catastrophic happened afterward. If anything, things feel better."
THERAPIST: "Good to get the feeling off your chest?"
MS. B: "Yes, it was. Scary, but worth it."

THERAPIST: "Perhaps *you've made things better*, by telling George how this situation makes you feel and setting a boundary?"

MS. B: "Well . . . I guess."

THERAPIST: It was brave of you to take the risk, and it seems to be paying off. Good to know you can assert yourself like that! And particularly good that you not only told him what you wanted, or didn't want, but also that you told him how you felt when he interrupted."

They discussed George's generally patriarchal attitude and how that had gotten on her nerves even before the stroke. They explored and then role played how Ms. B might further discuss the marriage to reach a more equitable balance. At the midpoint evaluation (session 6), which immediately preceded this session, Ms. B's Ham-D score had fallen to 12, the mildly depressed range. Over the course of the next weeks, she mapped out an agreement with George that he would respect her work space as well as some other needs. For example, she was preparing dinner for five every night in addition to working full time and keeping an eye on her high school teens' homework. Perhaps it would be nice if he sat in the kitchen with her while she cooked? Tensions between them markedly improved, and George occasionally even apologized when he made a misstep.

She was getting out of the house more for walks and runs, which felt good, but not doing so simply to avoid conflict with George, she noted. Ms. B had somewhat regularized her social rhythms, within the limits of the lockdown. Feeling less depressed and more socially comfortable, she was speaking to friends more often, and speaking more frankly about how the pandemic had contributed to marital stress. Some of her friends had noticed similar pressures. She said they were impressed by her handling of her home life.

Termination

Ms. B said she was still not exactly comfortable with getting angry, but that she saw its value, was getting better at it, and more openly expressing frustration in a variety of settings. That results had generally been quite positive, both at home and work, she still found surprising. She had spoken to her boss and told him that she felt cut off without occasional one-to-one meetings, "that it bothered me." He had agreed to check in with her biweekly, which helped. She thus felt more in control of her environment, at home and elsewhere. "You've developed a valuable new option!" her therapist said. "Yes," she replied, "it does really free me up to be able to say 'no' to people! And to tell them what I need." At the end of treatment her Ham-D score was 7, consistent with remission. She remained on medication but did not feel the need for further treatment at that juncture, although she understood the door was open if she again felt worse. She recognized that her marriage was not going to be what she had envisioned before the stroke, which now made her sad, tearful at times, but not depressed. She ended therapy by thanking the therapist and saying, "I wish we had met in person. I would like to give you a hug." The therapist said: "It's been great working with you, and impressive to see how well you've handled a really difficult situation at a truly difficult time. I'll miss working with you, too."

ROLE TRANSITION

Mr. C, a 31-year-old single Catholic gay Hispanic actor, presented by Zoom for an evaluation with the chief complaint: "I'm really depressed." After some struggles in his career, he had gotten a break in a Broadway musical with a small but important singing role the critics applauded. For the first time in his life, he was approaching financial solvency, paying off considerable credit card loans. For the first time since college, he felt recognized for his talents. Pursuing a long-standing dream, he had auditioned for and gotten a speaking part in a summer Shakespeare in the Park production in Central Park, and had been very excited. He was outgoing, confident, handsome, active, a doer.

Then the pandemic hit. In March, Broadway went dark, and he found himself out of work. In mid-April came the formal announcement from the Public Theater canceling the Park Shakespeare summer season. Suddenly his career was in shambles. He was able to collect unemployment, but he felt cooped up in his studio apartment. He checked the want ads, but it seemed clear that theater would be shut down for some time. With bars and restaurants closed, his friends in isolation, his whole world turned upside down. He had been dating another, closeted actor, Hank, who went home to his family in a different state, where he came down with Covid-19. This put Mr. C into a state of "long-distance panic." He frantically tried to call his lover, but Hank was uncomfortable talking to him around his "white bread" family, febrile and short of breath, and slept a lot. Home alone, Mr. C tracked the news, spent hours on social media, and tried to binge-watch TV series and movies to distract himself.

He felt depressed and anxious, had trouble enjoying anything, worried his boyfriend would die far away and out of reach. He also felt he had lost his theatrical momentum and that Broadway might never return: his career, for which he had worked all of his life, was over just as it had been starting to take shape. Mr. C had difficulty falling and staying asleep, was losing weight for lack of appetite, and felt his life was over, although he denied active plans to kill himself. His mood was worst in the morning, as he awoke tired and miserable to face the prospects of another empty and frightening day. His Ham-D score was 31, severely depressed.

Born in the Dominican Republic, Mr. C grew up feeling loved and cared for in an impoverished, hardworking family. He was the second of four children and second son. He sang and danced from an early age, with his mother's support and his father's acquiescence. His mother was convinced he would be a star. When he was eight, the family moved to New York, where he gained admission to a high school for music and art. Mr. C had many friends, but most were social acquaintances, not people he really confided in. Similarly, although he said his family was "close" and accepted his sexuality, he tended not to talk to any of them about his personal problems, except *in extremis* his mother. He also noted that he previously had not had to rely on people: he denied any history of trauma, anxiety (although he had vomited before a couple of auditions), or previous depression. He drank alcohol and occasionally smoked pot, but such use had largely been social, not problematic. His family history included some relatives with alcohol and drug problems but no clear history of mood disorders or suicide.

Referred by a friend, Mr. C appeared promptly on Zoom, well groomed, good looking, stylishly dressed. His movements were agitated, his brow furrowed, his speech mildly pressured at first, slowing to a more normal pace as he unburdened himself. He made fair eye contact. Mood was anxious and depressed with a reactive, at moments slightly dramatic, tearful affect, but not really labile. He had goal-directed thinking with an impressionistic edge; he reported passive suicidal ideation without plans or intent. Sensorium was grossly clear.

At the end of the second session, the therapist gave this formulation:

"This pandemic has affected everyone, but it's really turned your life upside down: your career, your relationship, everything. No wonder you're upset when your life has been so upset. We call going through such change a *role transition*: you've at least temporarily lost valuable things in your life, and the present and future look uncertain at best. If you can manage this transition well, it should improve both your life situation, and through that, your mood. That's going to mean talking about your feelings about what you've lost, and your prospects for making things better in the present. . . . Does that make sense to you as a plan?"

Mr. C replied, "I guess. I just need help. I'm willing to try it."

Middle Phase

Sessions followed the plan laid out in the formulation. He mourned the closing of his current production and cancellation of his future one—acknowledging that it might be revived in the future, "but who knows where I'll be then?" They discussed what he could do while the theaters were closed, which led Mr. C to audition for a virtual theatrical production, where each actor would perform from home for audiences through a Zoom link. He didn't get the part, which was discouraging, but it at least kept him busy. Meanwhile, he was torn about what to do about Hank, who had not been hospitalized but was isolated in a bedroom of his parents' house. They texted intermittently—which is to say, Mr. C texted often, Hank on occasion when he was awake and alert enough to respond.

The therapist noted that Mr. C had many friends, but not many close friends, and that while he may never before have needed to rely on others, social support could really help in the midst of a crisis. Were there people he could turn to so that all the problems were not contained within himself, alone in his studio? What would it be like to do that? Mr. C was initially hesitant but then characterized role play as an audition. His first versions of what he might say sounded scripted and controlled, but on further tries he became more and more spontaneous and openly emotional.

He signed on to Zoom a couple of weekly sessions later and announced, in response to the opening question: "I'm feeling a little better, let me tell you what happened." In the end, he had opted to contact not a friend but his mother. He had not wanted to trouble her, and felt a little uncomfortable discussing his love life with her, but he did feel she would try to be supportive even if she didn't fully understand. He FaceTimed her, asked if she could speak with him privately, and found her immediately available. He told her how down and anxious he felt about the situation with Hank. She was soothing and supportive. (Thank goodness, thought the therapist.) Afterwards, he felt slightly uncomfortable but mainly relieved. And it hadn't in the end felt like a performance, but like real life.

This was a turning point in the therapy. He subsequently spoke to two friends about how he was doing. They, too, were generally supportive, and one gave him a lead about another virtual theater production for which he auditioned and did get a small role. It was essentially unpaid work, but it felt good to be back at his craft.

Termination

As the end of therapy approached, Mr. C looked brighter, calmer, happier. Hank was out of danger, feeling better, and hoping to return to New York, although the limited acting opportunities left him in limbo. Because he was well enough to leave his parents' house on walks, they were able to talk by phone more freely, and he expressed his appreciation for Mr. C's concern during his illness. Broadway theaters were still boarded up, but the virtual theater performance was approaching, and Mr. C felt that his career, although detoured, had not ended. Meanwhile, he was impressed that he'd been able to turn to people for support when he needed it, building interpersonal bonds that made him feel more connected to others.

By the end of treatment his Ham-D score had fallen to 6, indicated depressive remission (Ham-D ≤ 7). Mr. C understood that there was a possibility he could get depressed again in future, in which case he would seek further treatment, but at the moment he felt he had gotten enough from therapy and didn't need to continue. He asked his therapist to come see him perform in future. The therapist promised he would.

Mr. D, a 49-year-old co-habiting non-denominational African American sales agent, had been a patient in my practice for more than twenty years. He had originally presented with lifelong dysthymic disorder compounded into "double depression." Mr. D had done very well after a brief course of IPT mourning the tragic death of his father, a civil rights activist, combined with and followed by chronic maintenance on sertraline. In recent years I had regularly renewed sertraline prescriptions but had heard from him only when life became too difficult (often due to problems with his longtime, demanding fiancée, who shared his cramped apartment) and his mood dipped: this amounted to twice in the past six years. At such a moment he would reappear for a booster session or two of IPT. Mr. D liked to keep his feelings in check and to be self-sufficient. He called me in late June 2020, saying he had been crying for 14 hours and couldn't stop. We arranged a Zoom session for the next day.

He signed onto Zoom, alert, wearing a "POTUS = Nazi" t-shirt, his familiar if slightly older face looking tired and frazzled. He immediately began crying, which was unusual for him. His mood was sad, angry, and initially anxious, with congruent, nonlabile affect. Thinking was goal-directed, sensorium clear. "Doc, you're the psychiatrist, but I think I know what's going on." Several weeks into the nationwide Black Lives Matter protests, one of the seventy-plus publicized cases of white policemen killing young black men had caught him up: "I think it's that he was so innocent, wasn't doing anything wrong, told people he was different— and they just killed him. I can't stop crying, I feel broken." He sobbed for several minutes.

The feelings he had about the police victim's death also brought back memories of the life and death of his father, who as an African American civil rights activist had been threatened and jailed by white police. Yet when he turned to those around him to talk about his pain and outrage, his mother told Mr. D that crying was weak, and his frequently unsupportive fiancée told him to get over it, get with the program, enough is enough. This negative feedback reinforced his own sense that he needed to get his work done and that these unhelpful feelings were interfering.

We discussed how he should feel in the setting of such upsetting events.

MR. D: "Sad, upset."

THERAPIST: "Sad and what kind of upset?"

MR. D: "Sad, and hurt and disappointed, and it feels like everything is going wrong everywhere . . ."

THERAPIST: "So many terrible things are happening. Of course it's very upsetting. So what emotions did you have when you saw that video?"

MR. D: "Horrified. And I guess angry. He was innocent! [crying] There's been no justice for those cops. The DA covered it up, said nothing happened. Then the video came out, and seeing it broke me up. Unbelievable!"

THERAPIST: [after a pause] "It is! . . . And are those normal and under-standable reactions, sadness, hurt, disappointment, horror, and anger, to watching a young man murdered for no reason?"

MR. D: "Of course they are."

I said,

"I haven't seen you often lately, but I think I know you pretty well, and we've talked before about how you like to stay in control of your feelings. You haven't wanted to show people when you're down, and you're sensitized to those painful feelings and might want to avoid them. But as we've discussed in the past, sometimes feelings are helpful guides. If something this terrible happens, how terrible should you feel?"

It emerged that Mr. D, although avoiding the crowds of protests because of a heightened medical risk, had been active online in disseminating Black Lives Matter petitions, and the previous night had attended in person a musical vigil for the victim on the video. "I just started crying, I couldn't help it." He sobbed for a minute or longer. "It's very sad. Do people cry at funerals?" I asked. "Yes, of course, and now that you say that, I probably wasn't the only one there who cried."

In the course of this sad session, Mr. D denied neurovegetative symptoms aside from difficulty falling asleep on nights when he felt choked up by the injustice of events. We discussed the usual pandemic parameters: creating a structured schedule while working at home, including a regular sleep schedule; the need to get out of the claustrophobic studio for socially distanced, masked walks to avoid cabin fever; the importance of limiting social media exposure. At the same time social supports, including through social media, seemed crucial: Why not share these feelings with the many others who felt the same way?

We concluded that Mr. D was not having a depressive recurrence, but was appropriately upset; was not "broken," although perhaps the world he was reacting to was. The problem was the context, not something within. "I'm glad you're telling me I'm not crazy," he said, "and yes, the world is." "I'm sorry you're so upset, but I'm also not sorry," I replied. "You should be upset. You have every reason to be horrified, sad, and angry." I encouraged him to keep crying and remaining upset for as long as it felt right. He didn't want, and couldn't afford, further treatment at present, but we agreed that he would call me periodically to check in, and for an appointment the next time things felt out of control.

Comment

This is a not unusual example of the stress of the pandemic evoking such strong feelings that patients worry they are having a reactivation or recurrence of symptoms. Sometimes that is indeed the case, but often they simply need reassurance that it's normal to have powerful feelings in provoking times. It's important to contextualize the problem as external, not internal. There seemed no need for a medication adjustment—indeed, that might have given the wrong signal about the appropriateness of his emotional response. The story also illustrates the ongoing benefit of IPT in having helped this chronically depressed patient become aware of his feelings and emotional patterns.

There are moments when a therapist should maintain a certain neutrality, particularly on political issues—but this did not seem to be one of them. Having known this patient for many years, understanding his family background, and sharing many of his views, I felt this was a moment for solidarity.

Note that a successful IPT outcome benefits the patient at several levels. (1) It relieves the depressive syndrome: the patient feels better. (2) It does so by enabling the patient to better handle his or her environment, improving the patient's living situation and reducing external stressors.[70] This generally involves (3) learning new or improving old social skills, such as self-assertion or expressing anger in confronting the behavior of others, which many patients have previously found hard to do, and (4) understanding the benefits of and mobilizing social support. (5) On a more basic level, IPT seems at least partly to work through and improve self-reflection, leaving the patient with a deeper understanding of the meaning and utility of feelings the patient may previously have regarded as "bad" or weak.[70,95] For patients presenting in distress in the midst of or aftermath of a disaster, it builds self-confidence to be able to do all of this at a time of extreme, global stress. IPT helps patients adjust both to the crises in their environments and to the emotional turmoil this provokes within.

6

Posttraumatic Stress

It requires suffering a "Criterion A" trauma to meet criteria for PTSD. In this pandemic, many people have experienced severe stressors amounting to traumas. Some have weathered them without symptoms; others have developed posttraumatic symptoms without meeting criteria for full PTSD; and still others have been sufficiently traumatized and were sufficiently vulnerable to trauma that they meet DSM-5 criteria for the full PTSD syndrome. The first group, stunned but essentially asymptomatic, may well not need treatment; if they do seek help, simple support and reassurance may suffice.[103] Individuals who have subsyndromal posttraumatic symptoms may suffer and struggle to function, and may benefit from formal treatment.[104] Anyone with full PTSD (Box 6.1) deserves treatment, although these individuals unfortunately may take years to seek it.[105]

After a disaster you are likely to see two kinds of patients with PTSD or its symptoms: those with new trauma and those with reactivated trauma. Both deserve congratulations for seeking help: the former for doing so before their symptoms become terribly ingrained; the latter for recognizing the return or worsening of symptoms under the pressure of huge current stressors and for seeking help as well.

ADAPTATION

Because the diagnosis of PTSD demands a drastic life event, it would seem a likely treatment target for IPT, a life event–based treatment. The principal obstacle to conducting IPT for PTSD is that IPT focuses on the link between events and feelings, and a prime PTSD symptom for many patients is affectless numbness or severe emotional constriction. (Interestingly, whereas DSM-IV PTSD criteria included "restricted range of affect," the DSM-5 criterion set lacks this crucial symptom, while retaining symptoms C.1 and D.6 and D.7 [see Box 6.1].) Thus when you open a session with, "How have things been since we last met?" patients with PTSD invariably reply with an event, not a mood: "I almost got into a fight in a drug store." If you ask, "And what were you feeling when that happened?" the answer is often something like: "Nothing." "I don't know." "I didn't feel anything."[3]

Box 6.1:

DSM-5 Posttraumatic Stress Disorder (ICD Code F43.10)

A. **Exposure to actual or threatened death, serious injury, or sexual violence in one (or more) of the following ways:**
   1. Directly experiencing the traumatic event(s).
   2. Witnessing, in person, the event(s) as it occurred to others.
   3. Learning that the traumatic event(s) occurred to a close family member or close friend. In cases of actual or threatened death of family member or friend, the event(s) must have been violent or accidental.
   4. Experiencing repeated or extreme exposure to aversive details of the traumatic event(s) (e.g., first responders collecting human remains; police officers repeatedly exposed to details of child abuse).

Note: Criterion A4 does not apply to exposure through electronic media, television, movies, or pictures, unless this exposure is work related.

B. **Presence of one (or more) of the following intrusion symptoms associated with the traumatic event(s), beginning after the traumatic event(s) occurred:**
   1. Recurrent, involuntary, and intrusive distressing memories of the traumatic event(s).

Note: In children older than s years, repetitive play may occur in which themes or aspects of the traumatic event(s) are expressed.

   2. Recurrent distressing dreams in which the content and/or affect of the dream are related to the traumatic event(s).

Note: In children, there may be frightening dreams without recognizable content.

   3. Dissociative reactions (e.g., flashbacks) in which the individual feels or acts as if the traumatic event(s) were recurring. (Such reactions may occur on a continuum, with the most extreme expression being a complete loss of awareness of present surroundings.)

Note: In children, trauma-specific reenactment may occur in play.

   4. Intense or prolonged psychological distress at exposure to internal or external cues that symbolize or resemble an aspect of the traumatic event(s).
   5. Marked psychological reactions to internal or external cues that symbolize or resemble an aspect of the traumatic event(s).

C. **Persistent avoidance of stimuli associated with the traumatic event(s), beginning after the traumatic event(s) occurred, as evidenced by one or both of the following:**
   1. Avoidance of or efforts to avoid distressing memories, thoughts, or feelings about or closely associated with the traumatic event(s).
   2. Avoidance of or efforts to avoid external reminders (people, places, conversations, activities, objects, situations) that arouse distressing memories, thoughts, or feelings about or closely associated with the traumatic event(s).

D. **Negative alterations in cognitions and mood associated with the traumatic event(s), beginning or worsening after the traumatic event(s) occurred, as evidenced by two (or more) of the following:**
   1. Inability to remember an important aspect of the traumatic event(s) (typically due to dissociative amnesia and not to other factors such as head injury, alcohol, or drugs).
   2. Persistent and exaggerated negative beliefs or expectations about oneself, others, or the world (e.g., "I am bad," "No one can be trusted," "The world is completely dangerous," "My whole nervous system is permanently ruined").
   3. Persistent, distorted cognitions about the cause or consequences of the traumatic event(s) that lead the individual to blame himself/herself or others.
   4. Persistent negative emotion state (e.g., fear, horror, anger, guilt, or shame).
   5. Markedly diminished interest or participation in significant activities.
   6. Feelings of detachment or estrangement from others.
   7. Persistent inability to experience positive emotions (e.g., inability to experience happiness, satisfaction, or loving feelings).

Specify whether:

E. **Marked alterations in arousal and reactivity associated with the traumatic event(s), beginning or worsening after the traumatic event(s) occurred, as evidence by two (or more) of the following:**
   1. Irritable behavior and angry outbursts (with little or no provocation) typically expressed as verbal or physical aggression toward people or objects.
   2. Reckless or self-destructive behavior.
   3. Hypervigilance.
   4. Exaggerated startle response.
   5. Problems with concentration.
   6. Sleep disturbance (e.g., difficulty falling or staying asleep or restless sleep).

F. **Duration of the disturbance (Criteria B, C, D, and E) is more than 1 month.**

G. **The disturbance causes clinically significant distress or impairment in social, occupational, or other important areas of functioning.**
H. **The disturbance is not attributable to the physiological effects of a substance (e.g., medication, alcohol) or another medical condition.**

Specify whether:
With dissociative symptoms: The individual's symptoms meet the criteria for posttraumatic stress disorder, and in addition, in response to the stressor, the individual experiences persistent or recurrent symptoms of either of the following:

1. **Depersonalization:** Persistent or recurrent experiences of feeling detached from, and as if one were an outside observer of, one's mental processes or body (e.g., feeling as though one were in a dream; feeling a sense of unreality of self or body or of time moving slowly).
2. **Derealization:** Persistent or recurrent experiences of unreality of surroundings (e.g., the world around the individual is experienced as unreal, dreamlike, distant, or distorted).

Note: To use this subtype, the dissociative symptoms must not be attributable to the physiological effects of a substance (e.g., blackouts, behavior during alcohol intoxication) or another medical condition (e.g., complex partial seizures).
Specify whether:
With delayed expression: If the full diagnostic criteria are not met until at least 6 months after the event (although the onset and expression of some symptoms may be immediate).

American Psychiatric Association, 2013, pages 271–272[17] (emphasis in original). Reprinted with permission from the *Diagnostic and Statistical Manual of Mental Disorders*, Fifth Edition (Copyright © 2013). American Psychiatric Association. All Rights Reserved.

Thus, in order to conduct IPT it is essential to help patients reconnect with their feelings, which they suppress because the emotions to an overwhelming event feel so overwhelming. This suppression is something of a pressure cooker, and ultimately fails: anger will out, in the end, if often at the wrong target, which then confirms the individual's sense that his or her emotions are dangerous, unpredictable, not to be trusted, and need further suppression. In adapting IPT for PTSD, we therefore devoted the early sessions—sometimes the first half, if necessary—of treatment to *affective attunement*, helping patients to explore and recognize how they feel.[3]

The rationale is straightforward. Undergoing trauma can shatter any sense of safety people feel in their environment.[3,5] The world becomes a perilous, untrustable space, from which patients withdraw and in which they dissociate or depersonalize. It is understandable that anyone who has experienced an overwhelming trauma would react with overwhelming feelings, and some people find such feelings intolerable and try to bury them. But if you are unaware of your feelings, it's almost impossible to read your interpersonal environment and know whom to trust. Trust is key to PTSD and to having reasonable relationships. It's precisely through such emotions as anxiety (fear of an environmental threat), anger (sense of mistreatment), and sadness (sense of loss), as well as more positive emotions such as warmth, happiness, and trust, that we read what is happening in our interactions. If you're numb, you're at risk of revictimization. So IPT therapists tell patients with PTSD:

> "*Your feelings are powerful, but they're not dangerous.* It's better to know what's going on around you than to be flying blind. Knowing how you feel can be uncomfortable, but it alerts you to whom you can trust and whom you can't."

To achieve affective attunement, therapists gently push patients to tolerate and reflect upon their feelings. They need not—in fact, in IPT they do not—do this in conjunction with actual traumatic events but in the less charged setting of daily events. If a patient raises a quotidian incident, ask for the attached feeling. If the patient says, "Nothing," or "I don't know," sit and wait, expectantly. Usually a patient will volunteer, "I guess I was a little upset." But "upset" is nonspecific. You want to know: "*What kind of upset? What do you call that feeling?*"

Over time, in "upsetting" situations patients may report having felt irritation or annoyance—that is, anger, which is worth labeling as such. When you can help a patient to identify such an emotion, let him or her sit with it for a while. Inasmuch as irritation/annoyance/anger indicates not liking a behavior, or feeling mistreated, you can ultimately point that out and ask, "*Is it reasonable that you might have been annoyed when she did that?*" Over time, with such normalization of affects, patients learn an emotional vocabulary—itself a valuable outcome of therapy—and can begin to use it to understand and respond to interpersonal difficulties. Once the patient is affectively attuned, IPT can proceed as it does in the treatment of depression, helping the patient to resolve the focal interpersonal crisis (grief, role dispute, role transition).[3]

Anger is often a crucial emotion for traumatized patients. They may have been victims of excessive, abusive anger and have forsworn the emotion as bad and dangerous. Yet containing all one's anger over time becomes impossible: it leaks out in some uncomfortable fashion that backfires, leading the patient to distance himself or herself from the emotion all the more. Because anger signals mistreatment, it's central to the situation of many patients with PTSD. If they can recognize through their anger who is mistreating them and can mobilize the emotion to respond ("Don't do that to me! I don't like it when you do that"), they may modify the uncomfortable behaviors of others. Moreover, the response of the other person to such a confrontation may help determine how trustworthy they are. People who respond with an apology may be trustworthy; those who ignore the request not. Indeed, we prime many of our patients with this thought: "After he treats you like that, the very least you deserve is an apology." Many IPT patients with PTSD have ended up telling an offender: "You owe me an apology!"—and often getting one.

How to mobilize patients to take action in their lives is a frequent issue in psy-chotherapy. A basic, useful concept in the IPT treatment of role disputes is that there are some interpersonal *transgressions* that break universal moral rules, cross written or unwritten societal bounds.[7] Rape is always bad. So is cheating on a ro-mantic partner or physically assaulting someone. Having suffered through an in-terpersonal trauma, then, anyone has the moral right to demand of the victimizer, at minimum, a contrite apology.

It is useful to consider IPT for PTSD in the context of attachment theory and resilience. Social support protects against PTSD.[5] If you grow up with secure at-tachment, you are likely to have a trusting sense of other people and a broad so-cial network, certainly relative to people whose upbringing leaves them insecurely attached to others. If a trauma occurs, a securely attached individual has more people to turn to and a greater trust in reaching out to them, which means he or she will more likely discuss and process the traumatic event, dissipating its force. ("Let me tell you about the horrible thing that just happened to me.") In contrast, individuals with insecure attachment may have fewer (or no) confidants, and less confidence in seeking them out. Such individuals are more likely to avoid dealing with the trauma, increasing the likelihood of developing PTSD. In a pilot study,[13] we found that 14 weekly sessions of IPT for PTSD improved not only PTSD and depressive symptoms, but also attachment-related measures in treating PTSD in veterans. Interpersonal strengths may facilitate resilience, and IPT can facilitate interpersonal strengths (see Chapter 9).

In taking the history, the IPT therapist must take a careful trauma history, as patients once traumatized are often at risk for retraumatization. But having done so, IPT for PTSD treatment raises the issue of trauma only insofar as it is necessary to establish the diagnosis of PTSD, explain its symptoms, and justify the IPT treat-ment focus, which unlike exposure therapies is *not* on reliving traumatic events or facing trauma reminders, but on *examining the psychosocial consequences of having been traumatized.* This comes down to: "You've been through a terrible trauma. What has that done to your social life and interpersonal interactions?" In the context of the pandemic or another ongoing disaster, the effects of the disaster compound those of PTSD itself on social functioning.

Thus IPT for PTSD rarely touches on trauma at all beyond the initial session.[3] The interpersonal problem areas remain the same as for major depression, and they fit the experiences of patients who present with PTSD. On the other hand, the defining problem area needs to be trauma-related: for complicated bereavement, witnessing a *violent* death; for a role dispute, an *abusive* relationship pattern; and any DSM-5 criterion A trauma can alter one's life and life view and constitute a role transition. In our trials, role transitions have been the most frequently chosen focus (around 80%) of IPT for PTSD cases.[3,51]

In our pilot study of IPT for PTSD at Cornell University Medical College,[106] we arbitrarily chose a treatment length of fourteen weekly sessions, as opposed to the usual twelve for IPT for major depression. (The duration of IPT trials for major depression has ranged, somewhat arbitrarily, from eight to sixteen ses-sions.) Although it is unclear whether fourteen sessions is an optimal dosage, it has subsequently shown efficacy, and at least from a research perspective, we have since been stuck with it.

As in treating major depression—or any psychiatric disorder—it is important to serially measure symptoms to see whether the patient is improving or not. For PTSD, the preferred observer-rated instrument is the thirty-item semi-structured CAPS-5,[80] and the best self-report the twenty-item PCL-5.[81] The CAPS-5 is a definitive measure but can take forty-five minutes or longer to fully administer, whereas patients can complete the PCL-5 in five to ten minutes. A CAPS-5 score ≥26 or a PCL-5 score of 33 or higher is consistent with the diagnosis of PTSD.[107]

DIFFERENTIAL THERAPEUTICS

A range of treatments exist for PTSD. The best tested are exposure-based therapies, which are often effective but grueling. They require patients with PTSD, who spend their time avoiding reminders of their trauma (which can be ubiquitous), to face those reminders—that is, exposure-based treatment asks traumatized patients to confront their worst, most horrific fears. If they can face cues or enter situations that remind them of traumatic events, patients habituate: they realize that the fear-linked situations are not themselves dangerous, and their anxiety lessens. Although these PTSD treatments have the most evidence to support them, many patients understandably do not want to risk entering them, and those who do drop out at very high rates, roughly 30%.[10,108]

We conducted the only published study comparing IPT to prolonged exposure (PE),[109] which is the best tested and "gold standard" of the exposure-based treatments, and to relaxation therapy,[110] an active control condition. That trial of 110 unmedicated, mostly civilian patients with chronic PTSD found IPT was non-inferior to PE overall.[3,10] Moreover, IPT had advantages over PE for patients with comorbid major depression, who were more likely to drop out of the exposure treatment,[10] and for patients with sexual trauma.[111] Patients preferred IPT to the other treatments despite its relative lack of an evidence base (probably because it did not require them to undergo exposure exercises).[66] Among treatment responders, the benefits of fourteen IPT sessions persisted without further treatment at three-month follow-up.[112] Enough supportive evidence for IPT as a PTSD treatment exists from other trials[113,114] that IPT is now the rare non-exposure therapy included in Department of Defense/Veterans Administration treatment guidelines.[11]

If a patient with PTSD has had a single, recallable traumatic event, does not have high levels of dissociation,[115] and, most important, *is willing* to take on an exposure-based treatment, then PE,[109] cognitive processing therapy,[116] and eye movement desensitization and reprocessing,[117] are reasonable, better tested alternatives to IPT. Pharmacotherapy, usually using selective serotonin reuptake inhibitors (SSRIs),[118,119] and sometimes prazosin or other alpha-1 antagonists for nightmares,[120] can relieve symptoms but does not usually bring about remission.

Psychotherapy is typically necessary to help patients alter their traumatic mistrustful outlook, but pharmacotherapy can serve as a useful adjunct.[e.g.,121]

Case examples may illustrate the IPT approach.

COMPLICATED BEREAVEMENT

Dr. E, a 51-year-old married, white, Jewish Ivy League–educated senior ER physician at a major New York City hospital and father of two, was referred by a
consultation-liaison psychiatrist for treatment of PTSD. His chief complaint
was: "I can no longer do my job."

Dr. E. acknowledged that his career constituted an important part of his identity, that he was proud of his control of emergency situations, of "running a tight
ship" and being "cool under fire." When news came of Covid-19 and its likely
devastating effects on New York, he felt ready, and set up a meeting to prepare
his team. He and his colleagues petitioned the hospital administration for the
PPE they anticipated they would need. When the pandemic hit, however, he was
shocked. Ambulances constantly arrived with patients in respiratory distress.
Supplies of masks, gowns, gloves, and even disinfectants quickly gave out. Patients
died right and left. He was concerned that he might actually be spreading the infection when he and the nurses had to reuse PPE.

He returned home after extended shifts, exhausted and "empty." He showered
both at the hospital and upon arriving home to try to reduce the risk of infecting
his wife Julie and their teenage children. Julie, an ophthalmologist whose office
practice the pandemic had closed, tried to ask him about his day. Not wanting
to burden or scare her, he would just grunt, "You don't want to know." Feeling
"wired" when he went to bed, he had difficulty falling asleep. Images of the day's
horrific events—once, three patients in a row went into respiratory arrest—
made it hard to relax and sleep. He began waking regularly with nightmares
of standing by helplessly and watching patients die. When he heard of the suicide of Dr. Lorna Breen, another ER doctor, he retreated even more deeply into
his shell.

At some point in April he uncharacteristically decided to keep track of the
deaths of his patients. Some died in front of him; he knew that many others went
to the hospital's expanded ICUs, where the ventilator supply was inadequate. At
points he had to choose among too many patients for too few ventilators, feeling
he was unwillingly consigning the others to their deaths. By mid-May, his death
tally was over fifty. Dr. E's colleagues were outraged that their proud institution
and the government could mishandle matters so badly. He agreed intellectually,
but found it hard to have strong feelings about much of anything. He just wanted
to keep helping people, but his usual preparedness and hypercompetence were not
working. His colleagues noted that this usually confident and amiable man looked
dazed and withdrawn—so much more than even they felt, that they suggested he
seek help.

On presentation, Dr. E's PCL-5 score was 57, indicating severe PTSD; his Ham-D was 16, indicating mild to moderate depression. Dr. E reported mild depressive symptoms without suicidal ideation. He denied any prior trauma history or psychiatric history.

A superficially friendly but contained individual, Dr. E prided himself on his competence and self-sufficiency. In the past, he had enjoyed others' admiration at his accomplishments. He was outwardly engaging but kept people at arm's length. His interpersonal inventory consisted of his family of origin, from whom he was distant; his wife and children, whom he "protected" from the traumatic events of his days; several other doctors at work, with whom he had an occasional drink, but to whom he confided little about his life. Most of his other social contacts were his wife's friends: he got along with them but volunteered little beyond chatting.

On the Covid Checklist (Box 3.2 in Chapter 3), Dr. E had obvious concerns about Covid-19 infection, although he took great precautions and had thus far tested negative. His daily routine had changed in that he was spending longer shifts at work, approaching burnout, and was not sleeping well. He had never confided much in others and was doing less so now. He had no time for social media, although he spent nights on PubMed and medical media searching for clinical updates.

He called in promptly on Zoom. On mental status, he appeared alert but tired, with circles under his eyes and a crenelated brow beneath a receding hairline. With graying curly hair, slightly grizzled, looking older than his stated age, he wore scrubs and said he was calling on his laptop from an office adjacent to the Emergency Room. He moved with controlled agitation; spoke in unpressured, fluent speech; and made careful, consistent eye contact. His mood was anxious and mildly depressed as interpreted through a constricted, barely reactive, distanced affect. (This was hard to read on the computer screen.) Thinking was abstract and intellectualized: he recounted an excellent history, but the narrative seemed almost in the third person, as if he were describing himself as one of his patients. He did report some intrusive thoughts and images as we spoke. He denied suicidal and violent ideation, and his sensorium was grossly clear.

Based on Dr. E's crisply delivered history, the formulation seemed evident by the end of the initial evaluation session:

"I'm so sorry to hear even a fraction of what you've been through—what a nightmarish situation, and it's unfortunately far from over. What a terrible situation to be in. You're a hypercompetent doctor, you've always been able to handle chaos and emergency, but in this pandemic even you have felt overwhelmed—and no wonder. Under this extreme stress, seeing so many patients die, you've developed posttraumatic stress disorder, which is a treatable condition, and not your fault. As I'm sure you know, these are the symptoms. . . . There are a number of ways to treat this. . . ."

Presented with the therapeutic options, Dr. E said he preferred not to do exposure therapy and didn't want medication, except perhaps for sleep. They discussed sleep hygiene and containing his work schedule. He opted for fourteen sessions of IPT.

"You've given me a lot of helpful information—let me see whether I understand. You've witnessed such a number of deaths, and have felt so responsible—even though Covid-19 is an illness with limited treatment at this point—that your PTSD seems related to complicated grief. It's bad enough when you lose one patient, but fifty or more is more than any doctor can be expected to tolerate. And to have to choose who lives or dies—impossible. You've kind of buried your feelings. Is that right?"

"I . . . yeah." he replied.

"I suggest we spend the remaining 13 sessions focusing on the feelings this has stirred up in you and what you can do to handle them. If you can start to process those feelings, you're likely to feel a lot better, to be able to relax and better figure out a plan for handling this pandemic, and the PTSD is likely to recede. Does that make sense to you?"

It did.

Despite the therapist's presentation of medication in a medical model framework ("combining medication and psychotherapy is like taking insulin and controlling diet and exercise for diabetes"), Dr. E declined an SSRI, seeing taking one as a weakness and a "crutch." He did accept prazosin, however, rationalizing that he needed his sleep, didn't need nightmares, and could simultaneously address his borderline high normal blood pressure.

Early IPT sessions focused on affective attunement: when Dr. E described an incident at work or home, his therapist asked, "How were you feeling?" Although highly educated, Dr. E's vocabulary was restricted when it came to emotions, which he frankly saw as a hindrance. He was hesitant to address them at first: "If I focus on my feelings, they may interfere with my work. They never got in my way before, and I don't want them to now." The therapist pointed out that trying to suppress overwhelming feelings—in reaction to overwhelming events—took a lot of energy, and that he was struggling to continue to handle his job under the circumstances. Rather than trying to intellectually convince him of this, the therapist used the IPT paradigm ("How have things been since we last met?") to elicit Dr. E's feelings—which brought up not the medical horrors in the ER but his feelings about the rest of life. Dr. E had noticed that there was tension at home: that he was more irritable at home with his wife and children—as they had begun pointing out to him. On exploring this, Dr. E acknowledged being more easily annoyed, but said that what he was *really* upset about was the way the hospital was managing things.

DR. E: "Those idiot hospital managers, the Vice Presidents of Bippity Boo with their MBAs, getting paid more than the front-line doctors to fill out their paperwork—and they fuck everything up! Where are the masks and gowns and gloves we need? Why haven't they all been fired? Don't they care about other human beings? And I mean [care about] the staff as well as the patients!"

THERAPIST: "You do sound upset, alright. What kind of upset are you feeling?"

DR. E: "What do you think? I'm angry! Those two-bit, would-be corporate fools—they've been threatening to cut the nurses' pay, and you know they'll build in a raise for themselves, for doing such a fine job! I don't see *them* staying on past their shift to find us our essential supplies! They should be fired!"

THERAPIST: "It's scandalous. Is it reasonable to feel angry under such circumstances?"

Dr. E resoundingly agreed it was. Yet he had been holding the feeling in. "You can't say anything to them or you'll be accused of insubordination." His therapist waited until he had expounded on his anger for a good ten minutes; then noted, in the aftermath of this emotional moment: "Feelings are powerful, but they're not dangerous. They may hurt you more if you try to bury them. Of course you must be furious that these bureaucrats are hindering your efforts to treat people."

DR. E: "But what's the use of getting angry? It just gets in my way when I feel this way. Sometimes I feel like strangling those guys—which is a terrible thing for someone who's taken the Hippocratic oath."

THERAPIST: "It's a violation of the Hippocratic oath to *feel like* strangling them? [pause] It is upsetting, but you don't have a choice. When things happen that are unfair, when people interfere with your job, the reason you notice that something's wrong is that you feel anger. In that sense it's a useful signal. Feeling like strangling an incompetent is fine, so long as you don't actually strangle him. The question is, What can you do with your anger to get it off your chest? What options do you have?"

After a discussion, they role played Dr. E's giving a speech to his staff about how they should petition the hospital administration to get its act together. He was a little awkward with role play at first, saying it felt artificial, but found it easier with repetition. They rehearsed this a few times, until Dr. E—who usually prided himself on stoically not losing his cool—felt comfortable with both the content and the tone of what he'd like to say. "I want to come across as quietly and firmly outraged."

Dr. E's initiative was not assigned as homework. Nonetheless, never one to hesitate, he returned the following week (for Zoom session 4) reporting that he had written a petition, spoken to several groups of ER staff, collected signatures ranging from the doctors and nurses to orderlies and ER cleaning staff, and presented it to the head of the medical staff. It emerged that ICU personnel had similar feelings and also co-signed. The petition eventually led to a hospital-wide virtual conference and a promise from the administration to do better. Dr. E had his doubts about what this would actually accomplish, but he noted that he was feeling a little better, and that his family felt he was a little less irritable.

> THERAPIST: "Good that you were able to get that anger off your chest and use it in such a constructive way. When you address the feelings, they change. You may still be angry at the hospital, and with good reason, but it does feel different, doesn't it?"

Having recognized that not all of his negative emotions were so bad, Dr. E began to talk more about his sadness and helplessness in watching patients die, and in facing "impossible" decisions about whom to put on or take off an insufficient supply of ventilators. "They put me in the position of playing God, and it's been awful." Not being a religious man, he could take no comfort from faith. He cried in describing his witnessing the death "under my very hands" of an elderly but intellectually intact woman desperately struggling for breath, whom he gave oxygen but had no respirator to offer. Crying was extremely unusual for him, he said, but he noted feeling better, drained, decompressed afterwards. He spent part of another session recounting his feelings about the suicide of Dr. Breen. While he had never really felt suicidal, he could "understand where she was coming from. . . . She must have been burying her feelings the same as I was."

Patient and therapist discussed whether there was anyone to whom he could express some of these feelings. He didn't want to burden his wife with the details of his work stress ("She went into a practice where they avoid emergencies"), but he did have colleagues who he knew faced similar experiences. He met with a couple of them for coffee—carving out precious time in still frenetic schedules. This gave him such a sense of solidarity and support that his ER shift developed a weekly half-hour for (emotional) "debriefing." Following this success, he also opened up more to his wife.

The therapist and Dr. E spent a fair amount of time discussing situations in the ER: How much anxiety is appropriate anxiety? How much frustration/anger is appropriate? Dr. E at first wanted to "calibrate" this, intellectualizing the process, but after a time conceded that it "had to be a gut feeling." The therapist agreed and encouraged him: "Trust your feeling."

By mid-treatment (session 7) his PCL-5 score had fallen from 57 to 27, and his Ham-D from 14 to 9. He was pleased with these gains and able to attribute them to changes he was making in both his inner handling of feelings and his using them to handle external realities. In session 10, he asked to repeat the assessments: his PCL-5 was now 15 and his Ham-D 4, indicating remission. It was not so much that stressors had eased, but that he was addressing them directly and effectively. He had stopped the prazosin, which left him a little groggy in the morning, and found he was sleeping reasonably well without it.

Dr. E noted how busy he was and asked whether they could just end treatment after session 10. "It's not that I don't appreciate what we've been doing—this really changed my outlook on life, and got me through a crisis, I'm really thankful. But I need the time, both at work and at home, and you probably need the time to treat people who need your help more."

The therapist congratulated Dr. E on his progress and said that it was up to him when to stop. The therapist did suggest one additional Zoom session so that they could tie up the loose ends of the therapy and really say goodbye. Dr. E agreed.

In that final session, the therapist asked Dr. E to review *why* he was feeling better and how he felt about stopping. The doctor said that it had been revelatory to understand the utility of his feelings and to be able to translate them into use. He was feeling more comfortable with strong affects, more open in discussing them with others—"which really makes life a lot easier." He said he would miss therapy a little, "but you know me, I'm efficient, need to keep moving." He understood that he could return to treatment if he again felt worse, and he said he would need less convincing to do so. The therapist agreed with Dr. E's summary of his gains and congratulated him on catching the problem so fast: "Many people wait years before dealing with posttraumatic stress—you really took the bull by the horns." They had a warm goodbye, with the understanding that the door remained open and that Dr. E would check in in six months with a follow-up report.

Comment

This is an example of *de novo* psychiatric symptoms brought out by the extreme stressors of frontline medical work in a previously well-compensated individual who simply became overwhelmed by an overwhelming, traumatizing situation. The treatment turned on his rapid acknowledgement of his anger toward hospital administrators over their mishandling of his work environment. This is an example of moral injury,[18] definable as painful emotional reactions to "events such as perpetrating, failing to prevent, or bearing witness to acts that transgress deeply held moral beliefs and expectations."[122p695] Moral injury can overlap with PTSD, as it did here. Once Dr. E understood the situation, he showed great readiness for change[98] and made the kind of changes one hopes for in a time-limited therapy, indeed further compressing its time limit. He mourned losses, addressed changes in his hospital and home environments, learned new emotional and interpersonal skills, and marshalled social support.

Although the case report does not describe Dr. E's childhood and IPT did not focus on it, there were hints in his history of insecure attachment growing up under a disciplinarian father and a socially distracted mother who left him to fend for himself. He had responded with great intellectual, scholastic, and work confidence, but had always felt socially awkward, a feeling he covered with the bravado of hypercompetence. It was unsurprising, then, that under stress he tried to keep his feelings in rather than discuss them with others. He kept them in until he developed PTSD and felt he no longer could.

ROLE DISPUTE

Stress tends to make difficult situations worse. Ms. F, a 33-year-old white Protestant in public relations, presented on Zoom with the chief complaint: "I'm having a rough time." She lived in a cramped East Village one-bedroom apartment with her boyfriend of a year. "I got it for the nightlife, the location," she explained. She and Arthur had connected online and met at a Village bar. They had gotten along well enough that he moved in in January 2020. They both liked to drink, and Ms. F reported having had bad hangovers and a blackout or two in the past two years, although no seizures. She did not drink daily, but could drink a lot when she did. Arthur, eight years older and a former Marine, drank more regularly and heavily, and had been known to get angry and nasty when drunk, although he had never been violent toward her. Ms. F had mixed feelings about the relationship: she was getting to the age where she wanted to have a baby, but she wasn't sure whether Arthur was "the one" for her.

Things had gotten a little tense after Arthur moved in. She had known he was a slob, but he had promised it wouldn't be a problem. It was. The space was tighter than Ms. F had anticipated for the two of them. Arthur could be irritable. But they were getting along, mainly having a good time. Then came the pandemic. Arthur lost his bartending job in the economic shutdown; Ms. F continued to work, but remotely. The apartment felt still smaller. Worried about leaving the house and catching the virus, Ms. F tracked online developments in the news and with her friends when she wasn't working. Her mother in the Midwest left worried messages and phone calls checking on Ms. F's health in the Covid-19 epicenter.

Arthur, stuck at home out of a job, collecting unemployment, feeling there was nothing to do, became increasingly irritable and drank more. He complained that Ms. F was ignoring him for her work. The bottles began to pile up, and Arthur became newly explosive, at one point putting his fist through a wall and damaging a lamp. Ms. F, who said she rarely got angry and had never seen such behavior, was shocked. Arthur apologized, but thereafter continued to drink and became increasingly menacing. Ms. F, put off by his behavior, withdrew sexually. She wasn't sure what to do. Some friends said she should ask Arthur to leave, but he had no place to go and not enough money to rent a place by himself.

"Then things really got bad. . . . I don't really want to talk about it."

The therapist, concerned and expectant, watched her silently on the screen. Ms. F looked uncomfortable. "He did something he shouldn't have."

THERAPIST: [pause] "What happened?"

MS. F: [pause] "He had had too much to drink, and he got mean, and then he said, 'So what about'—having sex? I didn't want to, and I said it wasn't a good time, he had had too much to drink, but he made me. It was awful. I just lay there, waiting for him to finish."

The therapist felt like saying, "Shame on him! That's rape! Did you call the police?" but refrained, waiting to hear more of the story from Ms. F's perspective.

She gave Arthur the cold shoulder the next day and he, himself seemingly a little shocked, apologized. But it happened a second time, and a week later a third. Ms. F, now frantic, feeling trapped and threatened, wasn't sure what to do. She told Arthur this had to stop, but even she felt this sounded weak and ineffectual. She felt numb, depressed, and hopeless; had trouble sleeping including nightmares of being assaulted or trapped when she did fall asleep; and withdrew as much as she could. That still meant spending most of every day in the company of a man who had "turned into a monster." Life felt unreal, as if she were outside of herself, watching herself go through life's motions. She tried not to think about what had happened, but of course there were constant reminders.

This continued for a month before a work friend of hers, talking to Ms. F on FaceTime, said that she didn't sound like herself, that she seemed frightened and depressed. Ms. F replied, "It's nothing. I don't want to talk about it." The friend suggested that she get some help.

At her Zoom evaluation, Ms. F was alert, well-groomed as if for a job interview, but looked beleaguered, fidgety, and agitated. She was sitting on a bench in a fairly deserted pocket park because of lack of privacy in her apartment. (She had asked Arthur to step out of the apartment, but he had refused.) Her speech was fluent and unpressured, and she made good eye contact talking into her phone. Mood was anxious and depressed with a controlled, restricted affect, although at moments she seemed to be fighting tears. Thinking was goal-directed with fearful, depressive, pessimistic themes. She said life felt awful but that she had no plans to kill herself. Her PCL-5 score was 52 and Ham-D 23, consistent with PTSD and comorbid major depression.

The therapist extended the initial evaluation to nearly two hours because the situation seemed urgent. It emerged that Ms. F had grown up in rural Ohio in a family with an angry, heavy-drinking father and a passive mother. When she was seven and eight years old, she was repeatedly sexually molested by an uncle who threatened her not to tell anyone if she wanted to keep living. In any event, this was not a family where anyone raised problems or discussed feelings. Her father's drinking outbursts were studiously ignored and "forgotten" so as not to risk a beating. Ms. F was a good student and did her best to "get out of town" to college and then to New York, where she had built a small network of friends. She outwardly seemed confident, a façade she needed for her job, but underneath felt cautious about how much she could open up to others. She didn't like getting angry and "never" fought with people, seeing herself as more of a peacemaker. Alcohol had helped to loosen her tight self-control.

The therapist thanked her for providing so much information so quickly. "I know it's been hard to talk about some of this." He gave her her diagnoses with the formulation:

"No wonder you're feeling so frightened and depressed, trapped in an apartment with a man who's supposed to be a partner but is treating you so badly.

No one should make you have sex or do anything against your will. It's against the law, it's in fact rape. The first question is how to make things safe for you."

The therapist by this point felt great sympathy for the patient and vicarious rage at Arthur, but he recognized that displaying too much anger would only frighten this woman. He therefore pronounced "rape" with legal flatness rather than the anger he felt.

Ms. F, looking frightened, timidly agreed that she didn't feel safe. The therapist asked how she felt about her relationship with Arthur, what she would like to happen. She felt alienated from him but still felt she might care about him and was not sure what to do. "If he'd just stop drinking. . . ." She felt a break from him would be a relief, but could not envision achieving it. Were she to ask him to leave, he might get violent. Nor did she want to call the police. He had to this point abused her sexually but had not otherwise physically harmed her.

The therapist reiterated: "You have an excellent chance of getting better from these symptoms, but you need to be in a safe place to do it. How can we make sure that you don't get hurt more in the next week?" Ms. F thought she could ask her work friend, Ellie, if she could stay with her for a few days. Ellie shared an apartment and her roommate had returned to her parents' out-of-state home during the pandemic. She was a little embarrassed to ask for such a favor, having told Ellie nothing about her difficulties with Arthur. It was Ellie to whom she had denied trouble, and who had recommended her getting an evaluation. Ms. F also worried about Covid-19 infection in spending time with Ellie. On reflection, though, it was better than suffering through more of what she had been going through.

The therapist asked about contingencies: "How do you think Arthur is going to take this? . . . How can you handle that?" Ms. F decided on, and briefly role played, telling Arthur that she needed a break and didn't want to talk with him for a while. She didn't want to tell him where she would be staying. She and the therapist discussed responding to Arthur's anticipated angry reaction. This session was on a Thursday, and they scheduled a follow-up for the following Tuesday. The therapist told her to feel free to call his message machine or to email if problems arose.

Session 2 took place from Ms. F's borrowed room at Ellie's place. She had gone home, thrown some clothes and essentials into a big Fresh Direct shopping bag, and hurried out again, avoiding Arthur's questions and saying she had to go to the store. Ellie had come through "big time": she had been in a difficult relationship herself in the past, which had led her to swear off dating for most of a year. Ms. F was reluctant to tell her much of what had transpired, but what she recounted sufficed. She had fended off Arthur's increasingly angry and demanding texts, trying not to answer, just saying she "need[ed] a break." She also missed Arthur and being part of a couple. She was worried Arthur might damage her property. She felt that having moved out was a failure on her part. She had stopped drinking at the therapist's recommendation and was generally disgusted with what alcohol had done in her life. She wanted Arthur to stop drinking, too, at which point maybe they could get back together.

The therapist again noted that she had been through something horrific and in consequence had developed PTSD and depression. There were various ways to treat this, including medication, exposure therapies, and IPT. He explained what each of these entailed, and that medication could be combined with talking therapy. She declined the first two options, choosing IPT.

The therapist said,

"Okay, good. Look, it's no mystery why you're feeling so badly. The pandemic has been hard on everyone, but it's turned your relationship with Arthur into one where he's drinking too much, getting violent, sexually assaultive, and you're trapped in the house with him. You've gotten to a place of temporary safety, which is good, but obviously things are far from resolved. A relationship depends upon mutual trust and compromise, where no one gets everything they want but both partners meet each other's needs and respect each other's dislikes. In a relationship, you have to be able to safely say 'no.' That's not where you and Arthur are right now: he seems to feel he can do whatever he wants, and he's not respecting what you want and don't want. We call that kind of imbalance in a relationship a *role dispute*. If you want to continue with Arthur, you'll need to find a way to renegotiate things so that there's a balance you can live with. Does that make sense?"

Ms. F assented.

The therapist continued, "Let's use our remaining twelve sessions to solve that problem."

MS. F: "It seems like too much to accomplish."

THERAPIST: "Let's see how far you can get. You might surprise yourself. . . . As a first step, I'm going to ask you to pay attention to the feelings you have in situations with other people, including with Arthur, because those feelings will tell you a lot about what's going on and how you can react to the situation and have it work to your advantage."

Middle Phase

It had been evident in the first two sessions that Ms. F had distanced herself from and minimized her feelings, particularly negative affects. The therapist began to help her explore affective attunement.

THERAPIST: "How have things been since we last met?"

MS. F: "Things still are up in the air. I'm working from Ellie's, but Arthur's been bombarding me with messages. Some of them are a little nasty."

THERAPIST: "I'm sorry to hear that. Like what?"

MS. F: "Like: 'You bitch. Where are you? What's the matter with you?' That kind of thing, and I'm trying to be polite."

THERAPIST: "What's that like for you? How do you feel when you read one of those messages?"

MS. F: "Awful."

THERAPIST: "I bet. What kind of awful—which emotions?"

MS. F: "You know, upset."

THERAPIST: [silent, looking inquiringly]

MS. F: "I don't like it. I guess it bothers me a little."

THERAPIST: "So what do you call that feeling, being bothered?"

MS. F: "I guess a little annoyed. Do you want me to say 'angry'?"

Having let Ms. F sit with this feeling for a time, the therapist asked if such a feeling was warranted. She said it was.

THERAPIST: "Tell me what that anger's like."

MS. F: "I don't know."

But after further discussion, she did know: "Sometimes I'd like to say, 'Who are you to talk to me that way, big man? Who are you to treat me the way you've been treating me? It makes me hate you. No wonder I'm keeping my distance.'"

THERAPIST: "What about that?"

MS. F: "But of course I'd never say any of that to him."

THERAPIST: "Oh? Why not?"

MS. F: "Well, I never talk like that to anyone. It was just a feeling. And if I ever said anything like that, Arthur would blow up, maybe punch my lights out!" [Although she quickly reminded herself and the therapist that he had never actually hit her.]

THERAPIST: It was 'just a feeling'? Not a reasonable feeling?"

They agreed that she had every reason to feel angry at Arthur, and that she did not feel comfortable or safe expressing it.

THERAPIST: "What was it like just now, saying what you said?"

MS. F: "It actually felt pretty good, but it was just an idea."

THERAPIST: "Were you happy with the way you said it? Would you like to try saying it again?"

It was a tall order to expect someone who generally avoided confrontation to risk confrontation with a potentially violent estranged partner. Over the next sessions they discussed how she felt in greater depth; role played options for expressing her feelings and for addressing contingencies that might arise, such as Arthur angrily retaliating; and strategized how she might safely communicate. She had begun to respond to his texts, but quickly acknowledged that it was hard to make your feelings clear by text: "It's not like you can just add an angry emoji."

The therapist agreed that more direct communication would clarify things. She was nervous about FaceTiming, lest Arthur see where she was staying, so she began by phoning him.

Arthur was initially conciliatory on the phone but professed not to understand what the problem was. He wanted to know what she was up to, where had she been. Was she seeing someone else? He denied drinking, but at points he sounded drunk on the phone. Ms. F said something along the lines of, "We both know what you did to me, and you really hurt me, and I'm both sad and angry. I care about you and about us, and I'd like for us to find a way to make our relationship work, but we need to find a way to communicate where I feel safe, and feel like you're listening to me." When Arthur said that sounded okay, she continued, "That means you have to respect when I say no, including to sex. And your anger when you drink really scares me. You have to stop drinking if you want us to get back together. And maybe we need couples therapy, too."

That was too much for Arthur, who exploded as Ms. F had feared he would. Because it was on the phone, she listened for a minute, then hung up. He called back furiously and repeatedly texted her. She was shaken: on the one hand, she had said what she wanted. On the other, it wasn't clear Arthur could respond in a way she found safe. She called the therapist, half in panic but half pleased. "It's like I said it would be: he's ready to kill me." They again reviewed her options, including doing nothing until Arthur calmed down.

At her next session, Ms. F had come up with a new plan. She held the lease to the apartment Arthur now occupied, and she was also paying rent to Ellie. This didn't seem fair. She arranged to have a locksmith come to her apartment where, accompanied by Ellie and another friend she had informed of her predicament, she also showed up. After the locks had been changed, she said "no" to Arthur's demand of a key, and she and her two friends asked him to leave. The locksmith also looked at him shamingly. When Arthur protested, Ms. F surprised herself by saying (albeit she had prepared the line): "Do you want me to have to call the police?" Still protesting but abashed and flustered, Arthur gathered his things and left. "Where do you expect me to go, bitch?" were his parting words.

The apartment was a shambles, littered with empty beer and liquor bottles. Ms. F cleaned it up, aired it out, but worried that Arthur might return and attack her. She had previously discussed but rejected the possibility of getting an order of protection from Arthur. At this point she was still anxious, but also proud to have taken action. She simultaneously felt vindicated in her anger and afraid of retribution. Ellie agreed to stay with her for a few days, which was comforting. Ms. F now reported feeling better, and sleeping without nightmares, although she had a little difficulty falling asleep, listening for sounds that might herald Arthur's return.

She and Arthur tried again to talk, this time by FaceTime. Arthur was still unemployed, staying with his parents. He was adamant that he had no drinking problem and that he would never go to couples therapy. "For starters," she reported saying, "You owe me a real apology for the way you treated me." "I did tell you I was sorry," Arthur answered, "but you can't tell me how to behave." Ms. F said she valued him and their relationship that had been, but that she couldn't feel safe around him if he continued to drink. "Could you try going to AA, to see what it's like?" she suggested. "No way," he replied. She added a second lock to her door and scanned the street when she went outside, always with Ellie. They only saw him once, drunk, yelling at her from a distance—but he did keep his distance.

Termination

As it became clearer that things would not work out between them, Ms. F had bittersweet feelings. She began to mourn what she had lost in her relationship with Arthur. At the same time, she was relieved. She mused that he had seemed like an ineffectual bully during the locksmith confrontation. She didn't believe he had the motivation to cut out alcohol, and on reflection she was puzzled how she ever could have gotten involved with an alcoholic after having sworn to avoid her father's example in a partner. She also did not trust him sexually. At the same time, she remarked that a pandemic was a terrible time to date.

Her PCL-5 score had fallen to 18, which is well subthreshold for PTSD, and her Ham-D score was now 4, indicating depressive remission. Therapist and patient agreed that she had done a great job in a short time ("Without pills!" she laughed), and that while the future held uncertainties, she had gotten her life into much better shape and shed most of her symptoms in the process. She was much more in touch with her feelings and had figured out how to use them to her advantage. She was far more open with her friends. Her work from home continued to go well, and she had joined a socially distanced running group, exercise and socializing that made her feel better.

She was still worried that Arthur might suddenly appear on the street or at her door and hurt her, but that fear was both not completely unwarranted, given his previous behavior, and also seemed to be diminishing over time as he did not appear. "Perhaps he's in rehab," she half joked. They agreed that she was not completely over what she now called "sexual abuse"; she still shied away from the term "rape." Getting intimate with other men was going to be hard at first. It would be important to try to use her new emotional awareness and assertiveness to test whether she could trust them. Arthur had failed the test, but other men might respond better to her telling them what she wanted and didn't want. She rejoined dating apps and was half frightened and half relieved that Arthur was not on them. The therapist asked whether she had accomplished what she had set out to do. "It didn't turn out the way I expected, but yes, I did a lot more than I thought I could, and I'm feeling a lot better."

Even though she no longer met diagnostic criteria after fourteen sessions, she and the therapist opted because of the stress of the pandemic to continue IPT at once-a-fortnight frequency.

Comment

This case contains many of the elements common to PTSD histories. A history of childhood trauma, never processed and denied or hidden by the family, may breed insecure attachment, a risk factor for PTSD. Childhood trauma also constitutes a risk factor for "revictimization": such individuals often grow up with great discomfort about expressing anger, which can leave them defenseless when they most need it.[3,123] It often takes a lot of practice in role play to get it right, but patients feel greatly empowered and protected once they feel they can fight back.

This was a scary case, too, with an unpredictable, drunken partner the patient was initially unwilling to give up but came to see as impossible over time. The therapist was concerned about the patient's safety at several points, although thankfully nothing untoward occurred.

ROLE TRANSITION

Mr. G, a 24-year-old Hispanic Catholic male member of the National Guard, found himself in the midst of the pandemic assigned to morgue duty at a New York City hospital. His job was to move bodies from the hospital to the hospital morgue, and when that soon overloaded, to mobile freezer trailers that could contain the bodies. It was gruesome work, not what he had signed up for. He had enlisted to pay for college credits and stayed on because he wanted to be a good American. He had never envisioned having to do anything like this.

Mr. G had no history of trauma or psychiatric disorder. His family psychiatric history was unclear: no one had ever mentioned a problem. He came from an immigrant family and had idealistic aspirations for his country. This work, however, was grisly: carrying anonymous corpses, leaving them in trailers, worrying that he would catch the fatal virus from the dead. He had to reuse PPE due to a shortage at the hospital to which he was assigned. As the work continued, the experience left searing memories, provoked panic attacks and nightmares, left him feeling numb and dissociated. He worried and dreamed about the people who had died, about ghosts, and whether their corpses would infect him. He tried to follow orders, but he didn't find loyalty easy. It was typical of National Guard duty that he was assigned alone, without support, to do this work in an overwhelmed city hospital where the deaths piled on.

When he presented for treatment, Mr. G had a PCL-5 score of 43, consistent with PTSD, and a Ham-D depression score of 26, indicating severe major depressive disorder. His life had not always previously been easy, but he had never felt anything close to this bad. He was involved with a girlfriend, living elsewhere in New York State, whom he tried to shield from this horror, and who consequently had no sense of what he was going through.

Covid Behavioral Checklist (Box 3.2 in Chapter 3):

1. Mr. G reported great anxiety about infection, but it seemed largely warranted by his occupational task. He was obsessed with minor changes in physical sensations, fearing the onset of Covid-19. He maintained near fanatical hygiene and checked his temperature regularly.
2. His routine remained active, but the ongoing traumatic exposure was disrupting his sleep.
3. As his PTSD symptoms mounted, Mr. G withdrew from friends and family. He felt extremely alone in all aspects of his life.
4. He obsessively scoured the internet for Covid-19 information.

On mental status exam, Mr. G was a well-groomed Hispanic male appearing his stated age, with controlled but mildly agitated movements and fluent unpressured speech. He avoided Zoom eye contact. His mood was anxious and depressed with a restricted, nonlabile affect. Thinking was goal-directed, slightly concrete, with initially limited insight: he simply felt overwhelmed. He denied suicidal ideation. His sensorium was clear.

The formulation seemed clear by the end of the initial session:

"When you signed up for the National Guard, you could never have expected anything this horrible. When people face unimaginably overwhelming experiences—traumas—they can go numb and develop posttraumatic stress disorder, and that's what's happened to you. It's not your fault that this has happened, you're just trying to be a good soldier. PTSD is a treatable condition like many other medical problems, and in fact there's a good chance that with treatment you may feel better in a matter of weeks."

The therapist laid out treatment options including exposure therapies, pharmacotherapy, and IPT. Mr. G was willing to take an SSRI and prazosin, and asked for IPT. The therapist then continued:

"Going through anything like having to dispose of the bodies of Covid-19 patients is what we call a *role transition*: it's a major event that shakes up your sense of your life, and perhaps even your sense of who you feel you are. Your life feels out of control, as you've described, but it's really just a transition, a very upsetting change. As you understand and figure out ways to adjust to the change, you are likely to feel better. In a way, you need to mourn what you've lost by this experience; and also figure out what you may have gained, although that may be harder to see at the moment. Does that make sense to you?"

"Sort of. I think so," Mr. G replied. "I'm willing to try."

"Then let's use the remaining thirteen weeks of treatment trying to come up with ways to handle the impossible situation you're going through. I can understand your wanting to shut off your feelings at a time like this, but I'm actually going to encourage you to pay attention to them, because they're a guide to what's going on."

They also discussed basic sleep hygiene and regulating his sleep cycle; moderating online time; and the idea of social supports being helpful at such a stressful time.

In the next two sessions Mr. G reported continuing to be "freaked" by carrying bodies to the morgue. He was tolerating the medication and sleeping better, and he was starting to report his feelings in social interactions at the hospital. He had not reached out to civilian friends or family, feeling they wouldn't understand, but he had, after role play, called a fellow National Guardsman stationed elsewhere to commiserate, and that had felt pretty good.

The following week he did not appear for his Zoom appointment, nor did he respond to email or a phone message. The therapist was concerned and a little surprised: it had seemed clear that Mr. G, once he had taken on a task, would be determined to see it through. A week and a half later, Mr. G emailed to say that he had himself tested positive for Covid-19, had been hospitalized, but thankfully had not needed a respirator and was starting to recover. He and the therapist arranged a session for the next day.

Mr. G called promptly but was initially numb again, the way he had initially presented, and having lost the slight gains of the previous session. As it would have been ludicrous to ask, "How have things been . . . ?" the therapist said: "I'm so glad to hear from you again. Tell me what's happened!" Mr. G recounted having developed a fever and feeling short of breath after he had thought that his reused protective mask slipped in the morgue. His nasal swab had tested positive for Covid-19, and he ended up being admitted to the very hospital where he had been working. He was petrified: feeling physically ill, more than a little delirious in retrospect, and certain that he would be one of the next bodies to be transported. He had limited memories about a few febrile days, but it had been gratifying that the hospital staff recognized him as one of their own. One of his nurses had announced, "You're going to get special treatment here." He got better slowly, feeling supported in the process.

Describing this, Mr. G suddenly burst into tears—then quickly apologized. "It's okay to have strong feelings," said the therapist. "What just made you feel like crying?"

"It's—a lot of feelings," he replied. "I was scared to death I was going to die. And I felt really cared for by the hospital staff, like they were really on my side. I had been feeling so cut off and alone, but they made me feel like part of the team."

The therapist nodded to him on the screen but said nothing, letting the emotions unfold. It was a draining session. Mr. G said, "I know I'll have a headache after this." But he also looked relieved, and smiled at the session's end.

In subsequent sessions, Mr. G seemed much more relaxed, less anxious, as if he had decompressed. Physically recovered from Covid-19, he started back to work at his morgue assignment, which was still gruesome and distressing but no longer carried the risk of lethal infection: "I've got the antibodies now." He was reaching out more to family and friends, although he was concerned he not overburden them and omitted the gory details of his work. "Life is still a nightmare, but it's better to feel I'm not going it alone," he said. He was still somewhat anxious, but not panicky as he had weeks earlier. His affect was much fuller, and he seemed more comfortable with his feelings.

Termination

By the end of treatment, Mr. G said he felt "almost back to normal," improvement reflected in his PCL-5 score of 19 and Ham-D of 7. He attributed much of this improvement to the medication, which he had tolerated well. He was willing to continue the SSRI but had stopped the prazosin as his symptoms receded. The therapist agreed that the medication might have made an important difference, and encouraged him to continue the SSRI for at least six months. But the therapist also emphasized that Mr. G had taken charge of an overwhelming situation and made the best of it. "You deserve a medal," he said. Mr. G acknowledged being a "survivor, and I'm stronger for it." He noted greater tolerance of his emotions. There was the happy prospect of transfer to a different Guard assignment. He was back in close touch with his girlfriend and his family. He had a virtual beer party with National Guard colleagues on other posts. He thanked the therapist for his help, and said he'd miss their talks, but didn't feel he needed more treatment at this point. The therapist agreed.

Comment

This patient without prior psychopathology developed symptoms under devastating circumstances. Despite his symptom load, he was clearly motivated to make life changes, and he accomplished his mission.

Patients with PTSD have by definition been through horrible things. They can look and in fact be highly scarred by their traumas. Yet these patients often show amazing resilience in recovering from inconceivably bad events. This gives them a sense of survivorship, and often makes them look heroic—something you can tell your patient at the end of a successful treatment.

7

Anxiety and Other Distressing Symptoms

Depression and PTSD are two of the most common but far from the only psychiatric sequelae of trauma. Like those disorders, other diagnoses can either arise for the first time—for example, the initial onset of panic attacks—or can recur under the stress in the setting of disaster. IPT has been less well studied for anxiety disorders than for mood disorders, and the evidence is less compelling than it has been so far for mood disorders and PTSD. Nonetheless, existing research suggests IPT benefits patients with anxiety disorders such as panic and social anxiety,[72] and the typical interpersonal paradigm certainly appears to fit the presentations of patients with such disorders. A disaster provides a plausible context for the IPT stress diathesis model: under such circumstances, it is understandable to feel anxious or dysphoric. Patients presenting with subsyndromal symptoms still suffer but will likely be easier to treat: if IPT works for the full syndromes, it is likely to help less symptomatic patients as well.

ADAPTATIONS

The IPT approach is "transdiagnostic": it remains much the same no matter what the target. Of course it matters that you as a clinician have some familiarity with the target disorder, recognizing the symptoms and knowing what patterns to expect. That said, the goal is to link symptoms to life circumstances. For example, patients with panic disorder have a PTSD-like disconnection from strong negative emotions such as anger, which helps explain why their panic attacks seem to them to have come "out of the blue." It is therefore enlightening to help patients see that panic typically has an interpersonal trigger.[97] If someone in the environment does something threatening or enraging or otherwise upsetting, the patient may ignore it in the moment but then have an unexpected, uncomfortable explosion of affect later on. Similarly, binge-eating episodes of eating disorders are not random, but usually a reaction to some life stressor. In each case, the IPT approach is to help the patient to understand emotional reactions to daily life circumstances, to recognize those emotions as uncomfortable but useful interpersonal signals, and to help them find more adaptive (usually verbal) options for expressing them. This improves interpersonal functioning, makes the environment more hospitable, and relieves symptoms.

The challenge in gauging anxiety during a disaster is: how anxious ought one to be? Some anxiety is appropriate and salutary as a signal of threat. Some anxiety in social settings seems appropriate to social distancing, whereas when this reaches the level of social anxiety disorder, it's a disorder. Handwashing is protective hygiene; obsessive-compulsive disorder is excessive. Panic attacks and generalized anxiety disorder are clearly symptomatic excess.

DIFFERENTIAL THERAPEUTICS

There have not been enough trials to clarify how IPT compares to CBT,[72] which has been the mainstay of anxiety treatment, or to efficacious psychodynamic psychotherapies such as panic-focused psychodynamic psychotherapy.[124] Nor has any trial yet compared IPT to psychodynamic psychotherapy for anxiety disorders (or any other disorder). Of the anxiety disorder trials that have been conducted, those that have shown an advantage for CBT over IPT have suffered from CBT-driven investigator bias.[72] Thus the jury remains out for lack of evidence. From a therapeutic stance, it probably matters whether the patient likes the idea of homework and focusing on thoughts, breathing, and the like, in which case CBT may be a good choice. If the patient is more willing to focus on circumstance, feeling, and relationships, IPT seems a reasonable option. Again, in the context of disaster, circumstance looms large, anxiety is prevalent, and relationships are often strained.

IPT has never been tested as a treatment for OCD, a highly internalized disorder for which it seems ill-suited. Patients with OCD should receive exposure with response prevention cognitive behavioral therapy and/or SSRIs.

OTHER DISORDERS

Individuals with prior psychiatric histories may suffer onset, worsening, or recurrence of symptoms under the stress of a disaster. When this happens, IPT may apply to the extent it is ordinarily indicated. For example, IPT has demonstrated efficacy in the treatment of bulimia nervosa and binge-eating disorders.[7,125,126] The pressures of a lockdown, combined with fewer opportunities for exercise and more opportunities to visit the kitchen, might lead to worsening eating patterns and body image.

Individuals with bipolar disorder, highly sensitive to diurnal environmental change, may face particular risk during the pandemic because of the inherent restriction in activities and social distancing. The social rhythms aspect of interpersonal social rhythms therapy (IPSRT) was developed for and clearly benefits this patient population.[9,15,91,92] While maintaining social rhythms and a regular schedule and balancing social support during a pandemic are important for everyone, the recommendation holds even more strongly here. Anticipating patients' needs has led to good outcomes for the bipolar patients I treat. One bipolar expert I discussed this with, Dr. Holly Swartz (who studies IPSRT; personal communication, June 24, 2020) agreed, although Dr. Joseph Goldberg (a psychopharmacology maven; personal communication, June 25, 2020) was less sure that the stresses of the pandemic affected patients with bipolar disorder more than others.

Other patients may present with subsyndromal symptoms provoked by the stresses of the disaster. Again, such symptoms are usually easier to treat than the full burden of DSM-5 diagnoses for which IPT has shown benefit.

ROLE DISPUTE

Ms. H, a 28-year-old married, white Protestant social worker, presented on Zoom with panic attacks in the seventh month of her first pregnancy. She reported having had occasional panic attacks in her teens, but said she had had none in recent years. She had been nervous but mainly excited about her first, planned pregnancy with Matt, her husband of two years, and the pregnancy had gone smoothly until the coronavirus hit. Now she was petrified. Her Ham-A[82] score was quite elevated, at 30.

Ms. H had been anxious on and off since childhood. She had had difficulty starting school when her doting mother tried to leave the kindergarten and had had to return home early from summer camp due to extreme homesickness. Her first panic attack occurred with the onset of menarche, which she found confusing, painful, and frightening. Her mother took her to a CBT therapist, who taught her diaphragmatic breathing and other tools she found somewhat helpful; she stopped going after two or three months, feeling better enough. Indecisive, she constantly doubted and second-guessed herself. She did not meet criteria for OCD, depression, substance misuse (she drank an occasional glass of wine), and denied other psychiatric history. There was a family history of anxiety and drinking: one of her sisters was always very anxious, and her father had had an alcohol problem before achieving sobriety a decade back. She was medically healthy, took no medications, and her thyroid function tests were within normal limits. She met DSM-5 criteria for current panic disorder and more long-standing generalized anxiety disorder. She was highly sensitized to palpitations, dyspnea, and muscle tension, and often felt on the edge of losing control. She felt sensitive enough to panic that she had cut all caffeine from her diet.

Ms. H reported a "wonderful" relationship with Matt, an MBA consultant who was very excited about their child. She reported "nice" relationships with colleagues and had a few good friends to talk to, although she was not really one to confide her deeper feelings. She avoided conflict. She took an extremely supportive stance in her role as a social worker, was always doing things for other people, but didn't like to fight. She denied past trauma and historical antecedents that might explain this conflict avoidance: "That's just the way I've always been."

Similarly, she professed complete unawareness of why she might be having panic attacks, aside from the pandemic.

Something in her blithe and cursory description of her relationship with Matt struck the therapist, who asked further questions. They had met in her junior year of college, after a disastrous relationship had left her demoralized. Matt was buff, bluff, confident, seemed sure of himself. He spelled out what their life would be like, providing a defining comfort that this anxious woman had rarely felt before. When they discussed the details of her marriage, it emerged that Matt wasn't always aware of or considerate of her needs, and he dismissed her anxieties as "dumb stuff." He did seem to love her, but expressed it in a didactic, directive, paternalistic manner. "Just listen to me," he'd lecture. She felt misunderstood at times but really loved him, even feeling unworthy of him, and so tried to "meet him where he was, because you can't really change people like him."

They had both wanted to marry, and he had largely indulged her and her mother's elaborate wedding plans. They had excitedly planned a pregnancy, following Matt's lead. Always sensitive to somatic sensation, Ms. H became uncomfortable as the pregnancy advanced: not only physically uncomfortable, with bad morning sickness and intermittent vomiting, but increasingly anxious and panicky. The quickening was both exciting and terrifying, and she was ashamed to tell Matt that she worried about the damage the fetal kicks were doing to her internal organs. Despite normal evaluations and a low-risk pregnancy, she worried about the baby having "something wrong with her," and about delivery being traumatic.

The pandemic arrived during her sixth month of pregnancy, greatly increasing Ms. H's anxiety. Matt's business basically shut down with the economy, whereas Ms. H's caseload increased, and she began to hear horrific stories from the community in work she now conducted from home. She was terrified that she would get sick and either lose or damage the baby. In close quarters with Matt, who became increasingly irritable with the lockdown, she found him increasingly critical of her anxiety, which she tried unsuccessfully to suppress around him. He initially just told her to calm down, but after a couple of weeks was yelling at her several times a day, sometimes saying things like, "It's not the coronavirus that's going to harm the baby, it's your anxiety." In this setting, she began having near daily panic attacks, the worst she had ever had. The therapist asked: "So what was happening when the panic attacks started?" Ms. H professed having no idea. But when the therapist laid out the timeline and pointed to the marital strife, she concurred.

Reviewing the Covid Checklist (Box 3.2 in Chapter 3) revealed:

(1) Ms. H was terrified of getting the virus and giving it to her baby. She was taking appropriate, at points possibly excessive precautions, and seemed at low risk of infection.
(2) Pregnancy and anxiety were both increasingly disrupting her sleep, and she now missed a work commute that had allowed her to get closer to her clients and to set a boundary between home and work.

(3) Ms. H reported having less direct contact with clients, less contact overall with friends, and found herself at close quarters with increasing friction with Matt.

(4) She obsessively checked social media for news of the virus.

Being pregnant, and in any event worried about medication side effects, Ms. H wanted talking therapy rather than medication. She felt she knew the basics of CBT and so opted for IPT. The therapist considered formulating the treatment focusing on the role transition of pregnancy and the pandemic, but ultimately felt that the marital stresses were central to the problem.

Therapist: "You've given me a lot of helpful information; please tell me whether I understand what's been going on with you. You're in the midst of your first pregnancy, which is exciting but also more than a little scary. Then the pandemic hits, which is scary, and throws your life out of order. In part, the pandemic pushes you into tighter space and more friction with Matt, who's giving you a hard time, which makes you more anxious; and he reacts to that anxiety by getting angrier at you; and that's when the panic attacks really started. Is that right?"

MS. H: "I hadn't really looked at it that way, but yes, that makes sense."

THERAPIST: "You've always gone along with Matt's wishes as best you could, but you're in a very anxious-making situation where it's hard not to feel anxious. In fact, some anxiety is certainly normal under the circumstances. Some of your worries about catching the virus and about pregnancy are warranted, and you're not going to be able to shut them off: you're supposed to be anxious in a threatening or uncertain situation."

MS. H: "Uh-huh."

THERAPIST: "So when Matt demands that you be calm, is that reasonable?"

MS. H: "I shouldn't get *so* anxious, I know it bothers him. But it's a point, yes: there are things to be anxious about. And he knew I was an anxious person when he married me."

THERAPIST: "So how do you feel when he yells at you to calm down?"

MS. H: "He doesn't get it."

THERAPIST: "No, he doesn't. But how does that make you feel?"

MS. H: "It bothers me."

THERAPIST: "And maybe it should. So you and Matt are caught in a situation where he's making unreasonable demands that put you in a bind. Instead of his supporting you, in a way he's doing the opposite—he's part of the problem. We call this kind of relationship problem a *role dispute*: the two of you are not getting along, and it's harder on you than it is on him. I suggest we work on this for the remaining ten weeks of therapy. If you can renegotiate your marriage so that the two of you understand one another and he recognizes your needs, your marriage will be better, the rest of your pregnancy will go more smoothly (in fact, you may have your baby by then!), and your panic attacks are likely to go away. Does that make sense?"

Ms. H agreed to try.

Middle Phase

The opening question, "How have things been since we last met?" invariably evoked either an anxious mood, the report of a panic attack, or marital discord. The therapist tried to help Ms. H link her symptoms to her situation.

> THERAPIST: "I'm sorry to hear you're still having panic attacks. So what was going on before the last one?"
> MS. H: "Nothing. Everything was okay . . ."

It would then emerge, however, that Matt had been particularly critical. It took several sessions before she came to see the connection between the role dispute and her anxiety. Although panic attacks seemed to come out of the blue, they in fact had interpersonal antecedents.[97] The therapist asked about her emotions when Matt said things like, "Cut it out already, the baby will be fine. You're only doing her damage with all this fussing." She felt annoyed, even angry, but she didn't want to express it. "It's just not my style." They also discussed how she thought Matt might be feeling. Ms. H felt he was likely worried about the baby more than about her, which again did not make her comfortable.

> THERAPIST: "So how do you feel after he says something like this?"
> MS. H: "I hadn't thought about it, but now that we've discussed it: hurt, and I guess a little annoyed."
> THERAPIST: "Are those reasonable feelings? Does it make sense you feel that way?"
> MS. H: "Well, yes."
> THERAPIST: [after a pause, seeing whether she had anything to add] "So what do you do with those feelings?"
> MS. H: "I guess I just put them away. As we've discussed, I don't like to fight. I don't like conflict. Why get in a fight? He's not going to change."
> THERAPIST: "He's certainly not going to change if this pattern continues. But you're getting conflict anyway. This is not a great pattern for the two of you to be in."
> MS. H: "No, it sucks. I hate it."
> THERAPIST: "So what are your options? What could you do to change this pattern?"
> MS. H: "I don't know. It doesn't seem like there's anything."
> THERAPIST: [pause; when nothing follows:] "There are always options, even if the situation is difficult and they're hard to see. . . . What have you done in the past?"
> MS. H: "I've just gone along with him. But I know what you'll say, that's not working."
> THERAPIST: "So what else could you do?"
> MS. H: "I don't know. What can I do?"

THERAPIST: [after an unfruitful pause] "How much of what you've said to me about your feelings in these interchanges have you said to Matt?"

MS. H: "Almost none. . . . As a social worker, that's the kind of thing I might say to some of my clients, so it's funny to hear you say it to me. Yes, it's a point."

THERAPIST: "Saying something is an opportunity to get the anger off your chest, which should be a relief; and to help Matt understand where you stand. What might you want to say?"

MS. H: "I don't know—I'd really rather not say anything, but I see that if I don't this will just drag on, maybe even get worse. I guess I'd want to say: 'Matt, I love you but you really don't understand me. I'm freaking out about the baby, the delivery, the pandemic—but maybe even more that you don't seem to understand what I'm going through. I need you to support me rather than put me down.'"

In truth, it took a few role plays to arrive at this version of response, but Ms. H said she was satisfied with it. She hesitated to employ it, but a couple of weeks later, Matt said, "You're always worrying! You're worrying more about the baby than you are about me. Things are really bad." She then responded, saying in part: "Matt, I do love you, and we'll both love the baby too. But you don't really understand me. I'm freaking out. . . ." Matt was initially surprised, left the room, but then returned to apologize and say he'd try to do better. Ms. H expressed to Matt that she appreciated his response, and that what she really needed him to do was to "listen and not criticize me. I need your support." He again said he would try. Ms. H was both surprised and gratified by this outcome.

Matt behaved more supportively thereafter, communication between them continued to improve and to involve real discussion of their feelings. In so many words, Ms. H gently asked him not, as she put it to the therapist, to "mansplain" to her. Ms. H's panic attacks subsided.

Termination

Ms. H had historical difficulty with separation, and therapy proved no exception. There was a hiatus for her delivery, when she braved the hospital, worrying about coronavirus, but emerged unscathed with a healthy, darling baby girl. She had thought she would need a C-section, but in fact managed vaginal delivery without great difficulty and without the anticipated panic. Matt came to the delivery room and provided excellent Lamaze partner support, which she felt helped make the difference. She felt strong and supported throughout the birth admission. Afterward, she remained anxious at times—she worried when breastfeeding got off to a difficult start, but it soon improved—but panic free. Her Ham-A score had fallen to 13, in the mild range. She still didn't love confrontation but saw its utility, and used it to confront her mother in a minor skirmish over visiting and parenting. Because of the pandemic and the challenges of motherhood, she asked to continue IPT with the therapist. He agreed.

Comment

Ms. H not surprisingly developed resurgence of a past panic diathesis due to a convergence of physical, marital, and pandemic events. IPT could have been conducted here as either a (marital) role dispute or (motherhood) role transition, but the focus on the former may have helped to improve the marriage more directly than a role transition focus would have. Matt's compliance when confronted, validating Ms. H's faith in him, made an important difference in outcome. Therapists are always grateful for patients' flexible partners.

ROLE TRANSITION

Ms. J, a 26-year-old Korean-American lesbian freelance writer with social anxiety disorder, generalized anxiety disorder, and sporadic panic attacks, presented for in-person treatment in early January 2020. Her chief complaint was "I'm not happy, I'm not living much of a life." When asked what would make her happier, she had no answer: eyes downcast, she replied: "I don't know." She just knew that this life wasn't worth living.

Her lifelong, excruciating shyness made it next to impossible for her to make eye contact, to talk to people without blushing, indeed to talk to people with any comfort at all. She lived a retiring, essentially agoraphobic existence holed up in her apartment. Between her writing and a trust fund she was able to maintain this lifestyle.

She had a handful of female friends with whom she went to cultural activities and occasionally out for a drink. Even with them, she maintained a distance, horror-struck at the prospect of revealing her worries and self-doubts to them. She felt they barely put up with her and felt sure that with any added burden they would reject her forthwith. Ms. J had an extremely low tolerance for alcohol. Once every month or three she carefully dressed up, applied heavy makeup, visited lesbian bars, drank herself into an anesthetized state of low anxiety and no inhibition, and would wake up the next morning, post blackout, in a strange bed. She never maintained contact after such hook-ups, which only confirmed her very mixed feelings about the discomfort and weirdness of relationships. She would swear never to repeat this pattern, and held off—until the next time she drank. She never told her friends about any aspect of this sexual or drinking life. She had never had an ongoing relationship. She could not recall having had a fight with anyone other than occasionally in childhood with her sisters.

Ms. J had been attracted to girls from an early age and said she felt "okay" about wanting to be with women. Looking at the floor, she said that her family had in recent years stopped asking about boyfriends, probably knew she was gay, and might even be okay about it, but she had never discussed it with anyone. She was a first-generation American, the middle of three sisters, from a very traditional Korean family in which feelings were never discussed. Her tyrannical father, who had lowered his career expectations in moving to the United States, had angry outbursts, often hurling objects at her passive mother. After these incidents blew over, the family acted as if nothing had happened. All the women in the house were extremely reserved. The father had not attacked the patient, and she quietly denied any other trauma.

Raised in Washington State, the youngest of three daughters, she came to New York to attend college, dropping out for one semester due to painful shyness in the dorms. Referred by her school health service to a cognitive therapist, she dropped out after three sessions, finding it both overly intimate and simplistic in approach. Her family then bought her an apartment near the university, which gave her needed privacy, and she spontaneously returned to class, receiving a degree in journalism. She stayed on in New York, making occasional visits back to the West Coast.

On (in-person) mental status examination, Ms. J was a petite, demure, carefully groomed and chicly casually dressed woman appearing slightly younger than her stated age, wearing carefully applied makeup and a single earring. Her movements were controlled and tense; her speech soft, hesitant, and rather monotonal. She avoided eye contact, looking at the floor or toward the office window. Her mood was anxious and mildly depressed, with a constricted, controlled, nonlabile affect. Thinking was goal-directed but she often paused, a little wary, as if gauging how much to say. She acknowledged having limited trust in anyone, but denied frank paranoid and psychotic symptoms. She had an indirect way of saying no: pausing her speech, looking down, and subtly shaking her head. She felt her life was not worthwhile, sometimes thought she might as well be dead, but had never had plans or made attempts to hurt herself. Sensorium was grossly clear.

Ms. J declined the observer rated Ham-A[82] interview but consented to the self-rated Beck Anxiety Inventory,[127] on which she scored 32 (severe anxiety). She met DSM-5 criteria for social anxiety disorder, panic disorder with agoraphobia, and generalized anxiety disorder, with a host of psychic and somatic anxiety symptoms. She did not meet diagnostic criteria for a mood or traumatic disorder. Although she clearly used alcohol maladaptively for self-medication and relief, she did not meet formal criteria for an alcohol use disorder, and she denied other drug use. Her medical health was excellent and she strongly opposed to taking medication.

It took three full sessions to arrive at a formulation for what the therapist considered a challenging presentation. He struggled to disentangle psychological and cultural factors, despite his asking Ms. J about them at several points. Her symptoms were long-standing and social supports were chronically lacking. As symptomatic as Ms. J was, it seemed clear that she actually contained her anxiety through avoidance: by restricting her life, staying home, and avoiding people as much as possible. Yet this was also inherently unsatisfying. In some respects she appeared a better candidate for CBT, which the therapist offered her as an initial choice, but Ms. J insisted she had seen enough of that approach in her abortive encounter with it years before: "Not again. Not for me." Pharmacotherapy was similarly not an option. From an IPT perspective, Ms. J's story could have categorized her in the interpersonal deficits category: no one had died, she had no dramatic role transition, with her life in fact stagnating. There was the suggestion of a covert role dispute with her family, from whom the patient conceded she distanced herself, particularly when it came to her personal life; but then she did that with everyone.

Rather than resort to the interpersonal deficits focus, the therapist opted to invoke an iatrogenic role transition.[101] The idea here is that the patient has had symptoms so long, she cannot distinguish them from who she is. The role transition therefore occurs in the therapy itself: the patient learns to distance herself from the anxiety disorder, to see them as symptoms, making them an ego-dystonic syndrome, and to find beneath them the healthy potential self she has never clearly seen before. This approach seems to benefit patients with chronic disorders such as dysthymic disorder and social anxiety disorder.[6,71,72,101]

The formulation, gently offered, went as follows:

"I know that this has been hard for you so far, but you've given me a lot of information about yourself. Please tell me if I'm understanding you. Your anxiety scores are quite high, and the emotional and physical discomfort particularly comes out when you have to deal with other people. We call this social anxiety disorder, which is treatable and not your fault. It is really restricting your life; it's really why you don't find life worthwhile: the anxiety is paralyzing and keeps you from doing anything.

"Part of the problem is that you've had this social anxiety for so long, you think it's you—you can barely remember a time when you haven't felt so tense and uncomfortable. I suggest that we spend the next 11 weeks working on helping you to understand what brings up the anxiety, how it gets in the way, and how you can fight it and make interactions with other people more comfortable. Dealing with people is complicated, but it doesn't have to be so complicated by your anxiety. It's helpful for most people to have the support of others, not to feel so cut off and alone with their feelings. Does that make sense to you?"

Ms. J nodded in assent.

Middle Phase

The austerity and emptiness of Ms. J's life made IPT challenging. She always came to the office two minutes early, sat down, and was silent. "How have things been since we last met?" generally elicited, "I don't know" or "Nothing's going on." Then silence. The therapist asked how she felt about this absence. Ms. J didn't like it, felt it was frustrating, "but that's my life." They discussed what made contact and especially eye contact so difficult. Ms. J felt that people looked at her critically, perhaps as an Asian stereotype. She always expected criticism, blushed too easily, felt people wouldn't like her because she had no personality. "No one wants a 'nervouser,'" she said softly. The therapist suggested that this was a good moment to take some chances, risking social encounters so that they could talk about what specifically bothered her, and to look also at the benefits of social contact.

About a month into treatment, Ms. J came entered the office a little less carefully groomed and looking hung over and miserable. She sat down and said nothing for a minute, looking disconsolate and embarrassed. Then, in a delayed response to the opening question, she said that she was feeling guilty and depressed. The night before had been one of her drinking and hook-up nights. She had gone to a bar planning to nurse her drinks so that she wouldn't have a blackout, but things had gone the way they always did. She saw a woman there whom she found attractive, but dared not approach her. She had a couple of drinks to build up her courage, at which point the other woman actually approached her. It was scary but exciting. She drank more. She remembered leaving the bar_—but not much beyond that. She woke the next morning too embarrassed, too upset with herself to talk to the woman, not even sure of her name; and instead fled, returning home.

This led to a discussion of what she wanted in relationships. She felt it was fine to be lesbian in principle, but had mixed feelings in her own case because her family would not approve. On days like this, she thought of her parents' disappointment with her. She acknowledged, too, that she had been avoiding her family because of such feelings.

THERAPIST: "So you feel caught. It's a difficult situation?:"
MS. J: "Uh-huh."
THERAPIST: "But really, there's nothing wrong with wanting to be with women?"
MS. J: No, but for my family—"
THERAPIST: "What about for you?"
MS. J: "I'm fine. I'm living in the twenty-first century."
THERAPIST: "And should you be able to live your life in the way you want?"
MS. J: "Yes. But I don't know that my family agrees. My father used to say bad things about my gay cousin . . ."
THERAPIST: "That's a dilemma. What are you worried would happen if he knew how you feel? . . . What options do you have to deal with it?"

After discussion, Ms. J resolved that it would make sense to come out to her family. They might not be as unreasonable as she feared, and in any case she'd no longer have to hide the issue. They agreed that this was best done as directly as possible: even though an email or letter (her parents didn't text) might in some respects feel safer to her, Ms. J acknowledged that there was much greater room for misunderstanding that way. They role played different scenarios. She was awkward, avoided eye contact, but gradually developed a coherent disclosure: "I'm gay, and I haven't told you until now, but I'm hoping you'll be okay with it. I don't want this to get in the way of our relationships."

The therapist didn't anticipate immediate action by this frightened patient, so the next session proved a pleasant surprise. Ms. J came in with half a smile on her face. She had not wanted to risk coming out to her parents, "so I started with my older sister," to whom she had always felt close. She was anxious and sweaty when she FaceTimed her, her heart pounding in her ears: "I almost had a panic attack." She had had to look away from the screen. Yet her sister was patient, supportive, and said she had been suspecting the truth for some time. "Whatever makes you happy," she said. The patient was relieved, and pleased that she had mustered the courage to say something. Following this success, she had spontaneously told one of her New York friends as well.

In subsequent weeks she told her grandmother, her other sister, and finally her parents. They, the greatest challenge, didn't say much, but didn't criticize her or make her feel guilty as she had feared. Ms. J's BAI score had decreased to 20, a meaningful improvement. She looked much less tense, was no longer reporting panic attacks, and seemed more comfortable with her feelings. The focus shifted to her annoyance with an editor she worked with and with friends whom she felt were ignoring her. The therapist worked to normalize her frustration and anger and again to explore and role play verbal options for expressing it. Ms. J had typically put up with friends' unwanted behaviors or made indirect, sarcastic comments, so a more direct expression of "Would you mind not doing that?" took practice.

Termination

As acute IPT was winding down, patient and therapist discussed what Ms. J wanted in the future. She was much less symptomatic: a week 10 BAI score was 14, in the "mild" range. She still made no direct eye contact, but now looked to the periphery of the face rather than at the floor. Her posture was more relaxed, and she spoke more spontaneously, if still in short bursts. Ms. J was getting out more, seeing her friends more often, and expressing herself better. She said she would like to try having more of a real relationship than in the past and had even been looking at online dating sites. In week 12, she reported having met a shy woman, Katrina, online: "Nothing happened, we just talked." But it was promising, and she was considering maybe seeing her for a coffee, even though that thought provoked more anxiety.

Continuation

The therapist had planned to terminate acute treatment after 14 weekly sessions but to offer Ms. J continuation IPT: although she was feeling and functioning better than she had been in years, felt better about her sexual identity, and had improved relationships with family and friends, she was entering strange new interpersonal territory and acknowledged her need to continue building greater social skills. But then the pandemic hit, and it seemed a particularly bad time to end treatment with a still isolated and anxious woman. The Covid-19 pandemic hit Ms. J hard. Going down the Covid Checklist (Box 3.2 in Chapter 3):

1. She was petrified of getting Covid-19. Discovering that she was at the national viral epicenter and the state lockdown reinforced her long history of social withdrawal just as it had seemed to be improving. She now went outside as infrequently as possible, spending weeks locked in her apartment. She was uncomfortable even taking the elevator to her building lobby to check the mail. She had food supplies delivered but was reluctant to venture out on the street. She purchased quantities of PPE, which she then did not use, and hand sanitizers, which she did, compulsively. Indeed, even though her further retreat left her at minimal risk of infection, she developed new, obsessive-compulsive cleaning rituals. Her BAI climbed back to 30.

2. Ms. J had begun to become less reclusive, but the lockdown disrupted her daily routine, depriving her of exercise by keeping her indoors. Her sleep schedule, always somewhat erratic given the flexibility of her freelance work, became still less organized. Her new worries delayed falling asleep, but she was sleeping soundly, for seven or eight hours, and awoke nervous but relatively refreshed.

3. Her social circle, tiny to begin with but having recently expanded, constricted with the pandemic. She spoke less to friends, feeling it awkward that there was nothing to talk about. She felt it was no longer realistic even to think of dating—although she remained distantly interested in Katrina and texted her frequently.

4. Ms. J had always spent a lot of time on social media, but this increased during the lockdown. Facebook had always provided "friends" she could talk to more casually than in past face-to-face or present Zoom contacts. She obsessively tracked both the virus and current politics.

Ms. J and her therapist agreed to continue weekly IPT by Zoom. They discussed the anxious reality of the early pandemic, the need to recognize and respond to appropriate fear while not overreacting. The therapist encouraged her to structure her life, to maintain social contacts, and to limit her time on social media. Ms. J reported that her own friends were as frightened as she was and did not want to meet in person any more than she did, even with social distancing.

As the weeks passed, her anxiety diminished. She said she actually felt more comfortable talking by Zoom than in person, even approaching eye contact with the therapist at times. She reported trying to maintain at least a texting relationship with her "date," Katrina. The two of them joked that they had met at a bad time, both of them very cautious people who waited for the other to make the first move; and now even more frightened at such a scary time. Because they lived too far apart to walk and both feared taking public transportation or taxis, they opted not to actually meet in person. Blushing, Ms. J confessed that even though they had not physically consummated the relationship, it felt like the most intimate one she had ever had. She was shy about telling Katrina her feelings, but worked on this in role play. Katrina sounded almost equally shy.

Ms. J became increasingly angry about national politics and a sense that she was being discriminated against. This sense of oppression stemmed both from her concern that she was perceived as "an Asian" indistinguishable to other Americans from someone Chinese; she feared being blamed for what the President was calling the "Kung Flu" and "Asian Flu"; and because she was gay.[128] Her anger, surprisingly overt to her, coincided with the groundswell of anger following the police murder of George Floyd in June 2020. The therapist supported her anger as a healthy response to racism. Raising her courage and speaking by phone to Katrina about this, she was shocked when Katrina, who was white, discounted her concerns: "Oh, maybe [there's discrimination] in some places, but it's not so bad in New York." Ms. J took this as an irreconcilable difference between them, broke off the call, and stopped contacting her. Katrina fell silent too.

Discussing this with her therapist, Ms. J recognized that she had been so shocked, she had not communicated how she felt to Katrina. As communicating her feelings had been the theme of therapy from the start, she volunteered the option of contacting Katrina, both to try to understand her precise point of view and to communicate both her own sense of oppression and her anger and disappointment toward Katrina. She and the therapist discussed the inevitability of differences in relationships and the importance of trying to work them out. She called, left a message, and texted Katrina as well requesting a phone call. Katrina did not respond for a couple of days, then sent a long text saying that she had thought better of their friendship and maybe they shouldn't talk. She apologized for communicating this in a text rather than the requested call.

Ms. J was understandably hurt, feeling she had cared more for Katrina than Katrina for her, and that this was a shabby way to end a relationship. She felt vindicated in her initial anger at Katrina's previous remarks. The therapist agreed. Ms. J did express satisfaction that she had at least tried to approach things in a "grown-up" way, which was more than Katrina had done. She felt sad, angry, and disappointed, but did not become depressed or panicky. Her BAI score again dropped to the low teens. She no longer went to pick-up bars—in part because the bars had been shut. She would like to meet women in different ways. "Covid-weary," she continues in maintenance IPT with the goal of finding a fuller relationship once the city "reopens," while recognizing that reopening was likely to raise her anxiety level about infection.

Comment

This is a complicated case with a generally positive if bittersweet outcome to this point. Ms. J clearly gained better understanding and use of her feelings in the course of acute and continuation IPT. After she came out to her family about her sexuality, her anxiety symptoms decreased, she became more engaged with and tolerant of her feelings, and she used them to improve her social functioning. In a relatively short time, this near recluse came out about her sexuality, which was emotionally liberating. She then began, very tentatively, to explore dating for the first time. Unfortunately, the onset of the Covid-19 pandemic produced a setback, but she seems to be rebounding from it, showing resilience. She recognizes that she has a long way to go, but she at least feels she is moving in a healthy direction. At the time I write, still in treatment, she is generally able to distinguish herself from her social anxiety disorder, showing progress through her "iatrogenic role transition."

8

Termination

We have already covered the basics of terminating acute IPT in Chapter 3. The goals of this phase are to prepare the patient to end therapy, if therapy is to end. Even if patient and therapist plan to continue working together in maintenance IPT, it's helpful to use the last few sessions of the initial time-limited treatment to consolidate the patient's gains and feelings about the treatment at the end of acute treatment.

CONSOLIDATING GAINS

As already discussed, many patients will be feeling much better than when they entered treatment, but they may tend to credit the therapist (and/or medication) rather than themselves. The role of the therapist is to point out how much the patient has often accomplished in a short period of time, and at a time of great suffering, helplessness, and hopelessness. The patient will often have developed a new emotional vocabulary, gained trust in his or her feelings, and put them to use in communicating wishes or confronting the unwanted behavior of others, thereby resolving or at least greatly improving the interpersonal crisis that triggered seeking treatment.

People feel better if they are confident in their abilities. So the question, "*Why are you feeling so much better?*" gives the patient room to reflect on what has happened in treatment, what skills he or she may have learned, what he or she has changed. In general, patients often have a better understanding of their inner feelings and their outer relationships, and have discovered how to verbalize the former to improve the latter. Termination is an opportunity to reinforce those capabilities so that the autonomous patient, feeling like an active agent, will employ them in future.

FEELINGS ABOUT THE RELATIONSHIP

IPT does not focus on the transference or on the therapeutic relationship except insofar as is necessary to foster a strong therapeutic alliance.[7] Nonetheless, even in twelve (or even fewer) weeks, therapist and patient often build a strong bond. If therapy is ending, it's important to have a good interpersonal goodbye rather than to avoid the emotions involved in breaking off an intense if brief working relationship. Ending treatment is a mini-role transition about which the patient presumably has both positive and negative feelings, and it's in IPT mode to find a way to comfortably communicate these. The therapist can certainly reciprocate ("It's been a real pleasure, I've been really impressed with how you've handled things"; "I'll miss working with you," if that seems appropriate), but this should follow the patient's lead, not precede it.

It's reasonable to ask a patient to check in in the future, both to give you follow-up and to give the patient a sense of your caring and ongoing availability. Respecting the patient's autonomy, this is a request generally accompanied by "if it isn't a burden to you."

FORECASTING THE FUTURE

If the patient is leaving treatment, what problems will he or she face going forward? How will the patient hope to handle them?

NON-RESPONSE

Again, if the patient has not meaningfully improved in IPT, the end of acute treatment is an opportunity to blame the therapy rather than the patient for the lack of gain and to consider the variety of alternative treatments the patient could try. The goal of therapy is not to vindicate IPT but to get the patient better. Frequently, the patient has gained some greater understanding from therapy, made some progress in relationships, but symptoms have simply not followed. Thus the patient has kept his or her end of the IPT bargain; it is the therapy that has not delivered. It is unfortunate that no panaceas exist, so that sometimes a patient may have to try more than one evidence-based treatment to obtain needed relief. Multiple options exist. The therapist's goal is to acknowledge the patient's discouragement but not let that disappointment prevent the patient from obtaining the next, hopefully more beneficial treatment.

TERMINATION DURING A PANDEMIC

A prolonged crisis that quarantines and socially distances the populace may not be the best moment for some patients to end therapy. Time-limited acute IPT downplays the therapeutic relationship (certainly relative to psychodynamic psychotherapy) to focus on outside interpersonal relationships. The goal is to mobilize social supports and find and deepen "real life" relationships on which the patient can rely. Nonetheless, particularly in a time of disaster, by the end of the dozen or so weeks, for some patients you may remain the sole confidant and emotional contact.

There is nothing magic about the IPT time limit: it is simply an effective device to pressure the patient to act to resolve the interpersonal focus. (The general twelve- to sixteen-week range was adopted to allow comparison to medications in randomized controlled clinical trials.) Once the time limit expires, you can feel free to reset the contract, which is what happens in continuation and maintenance IPT. Not every patient will want or need to continue treatment, but many may. Supervising psychiatric residents at Columbia and therapists in the Military Family Wellness Center[50] during this pandemic, I and they generally felt it best not to terminate treatment for many patients who had benefited and continued to benefit from IPT.

CONTINUATION AND MAINTENANCE IPT

IPT not only works as an acute treatment but continues to work as a maintenance treatment, delaying or forestalling future depressive episodes of depression even at so low a dose as once a month (see Chapter 3).[75,76,87] Patients with already recurrent episodes of major depression are likely to have a relapse or further recurrence without some sort of ongoing treatment.[129,130] Ongoing IPT provides the flexibility of switching problem areas to deal with issues as they arise in the patient's life.

One study of maintenance IPT for women with recurrent major depression found that after two years of ongoing treatment, patients were likely to have fewer personality disorder traits on the Structured Clinical Interview for DSM-IV Axis II Personality Disorders (SCID-II) interview, less likely to meet criteria for personality disorders.[131] This fascinating outcome suggests not that IPT directly treated personality, but that many passive, dependent, and other seeming personality traits reflected the chronic influence of depression, and gradually improved with ongoing euthymia and with IPT fostering self-assertion.[101] As a general recommendation, inasmuch as treating personality disorders takes years whereas what used to be called Axis I disorders often are treatable in weeks, it's best to suspend judgment on whether the patient has a personality disorder until after the Axis I disorder is treated.

The benefits of maintenance IPT have not been assessed for PTSD or anxiety disorders. Still, in the setting of a pandemic, and particularly for very isolated individuals, it seems like a reasonable approach.

9

Dealing with
Post-Catastrophe — Resilience

As bad as things have been (and at time of writing, remain) in this pandemic, most people are likely to be "resilient." The term "resilience" has been so over-used of late that it has gotten somewhat worn down, and needs a little resilience itself. According to the *Oxford English Dictionary*, resilience means "the (or an) act of rebounding or springing back, rebound, recoil," "a tendency to return to a state," deriving from the Latin *salire*, to jump or leap.[132] Its psychological application connotes the ability to cope with a crisis, to manage life stressors without falling apart, returning quickly to the status quo. It's the sangfroid, the coolness under fire we all want to have. Scales exist to measure this buffer against stress.[e.g.,38] Moreover, the term has come to include posttraumatic growth,[133] the idea that you can learn from coping with adversity and emerge stronger than before.

Resilience is more complicated and elusive than the above definition suggests.[134] Resilience doesn't mean that people have no symptoms or aren't upset under stress. It also isn't an either/or status: people can be resilient up to a point, and then not. No one is invulnerable: everyone has some limit of endurance when beset by overwhelming stress: think of Job in the Bible. Nor is everyone resilient: too many people will clearly be hurt and impaired by disastrous experiences, and will need our help to try to gain resilience and recover. There is some agreement that resilience can be cultivated, strengthened with practice.[39,134] Where does resilience come from, and how might we foster it in patients? How can we help people to bounce back, and maybe even benefit, from surviving a disaster?

Resilience presumably follows a stress-diathesis model: some people have genetic and temperamental advantages that fortify them in stressful environments. But environment is key, particularly early life environment and attachment.[135,136] Dealing with crisis means having to handle the stress of change and loss, and we know that a crucial factor involved in this is social support.[137–139] Social support, in turn, depends upon one's social network and ability to use it, and hence upon attachment. As we have emphasized in the application of IPT to PTSD,[5] an individual faced with a crisis can either try to go it alone or turn to people in his or her environment for support. That choice is likely to depend upon whether the individual has grown up with secure attachment.

As John Bowlby pointed out decades ago,[135,136] growing up with approving, supportive, and available parents confers great benefits. A child crawling or toddling into a strange environment may have a reliable, attentive caretaker who provides reassurance and praise ("Good walking! You're doing fine!"). Such a pattern, repeated over time, might well impart the sense that there are supportive people around you should you need help, encourages a sense of safety and competence, and leads to bolder exploration of the environment. This secure attachment translates over the course of development to a sense that most people are trustworthy. Trusting people promotes a thriving social network. Should such a securely attached individual encounter disaster or tragedy, he or she is likely to have friends and family to turn to and to feel comfortable in turning to them.

By contrast, children who have indifferent, overly critical, unreliable, unavailable, or abusive caretakers will not get the same positive reinforcement. They are more likely to conclude that other people cannot be counted on or are outright dangerous, and to feel at greater risk in new environments. The social support network of such individuals with insecure or disorganized attachment is likely to be sparser, and they are likely to feel less comfortable in confiding in those fewer contacts. Hence in crisis they will have fewer people to turn to, feel less confident in turning to them, and more likely be socially isolated.[3,5] They hence will likely keep their feelings bottled up within themselves, which may make them more prone to develop emotional symptoms.

Thus secure attachment is a foundation for resilience, and insecure attachment a risk factor. IPT, as an affect-, life event-, and attachment-focused therapy, fits neatly into this framework. We recently conducted an open trial of fourteen weeks of IPT for PTSD, treating twenty-nine military veterans with PTSD.[13] We assessed at several time points not only their symptoms of PTSD (CAPS-5[80]) and depression (Ham-D[78]), but also attachment-related measures such as separation anxiety (Structured Clinical Interview for Separation Anxiety Symptoms [SCI-SAS][140]) and Symptom-Specific Reflective Function.[141,142] This study yielded several intriguing findings. Among them, are the following.

First, prior to treatment, 69% of the patients met criteria for adult separation anxiety disorder on the SCI-SAS, suggesting that many veterans with PTSD have insecure attachment either as a risk factor for PTSD or as a consequence of their trauma. This accords with a very large World Health Organization epidemiological survey ($N = 38,993$) suggesting that separation anxiety disorder predisposed to PTSD following trauma.[143] Having separation anxiety disorder did not affect baseline PTSD or depression symptom severity in our study.

Second, the seventeen patients who completed treatment showed improvement not only in PTSD and depression symptoms, but in adult separation anxiety symptoms ($p = 0.009$)—even though this was not something IPT was directly targeting. Improvement in adult separation

anxiety symptoms predicted improvement in depressive symptoms
($p = 0.049$). Among patients with baseline separation anxiety disorder,
early improvement (week 4) in Symptom-Specific Reflective Function—
in effect, the ability to understand one's emotions—predicted later (week
14) improvement in separation anxiety symptoms ($p = 0.21$).

Our interpretation of these preliminary results is that IPT may work, at least
in part, through repairing attachment: helping patients who feel very insecure
and isolated to feel more secure and connected.[4,12] IPT for PTSD in particular
focuses on confronting other individuals to determine whether the relationship
is trustworthy, but the principle extends throughout its application across psychiatric disorders. By helping patients to understand their feelings toward others,
and the feelings of others towards them, and using them to manage relationships,
IPT may repair attachment, and therefore enhance resilience. This issue requires
further research: the study sample was small, there was no comparison condition
to test specificity of the approach, and we did not actually measure resilience as
such, but rather its proxy in separation anxiety disorder. Nonetheless, the study
findings suggest a plausible and useful model linking IPT, attachment, and at least
one aspect of resilience.

Posttraumatic growth, meaning a positive psychological outcome in response
to a trauma,[144] is an appealing idea: finding a thundercloud's silver lining, turning
lemons into lemonade. It has sometimes been applied simplistically. When
patients present posttrauma for treatment, they are suffering. They tend to see
little or nothing positive in their situation. Therapists should take care not to
oversell posttraumatic growth, in effect cheerily characterizing trauma as a good
thing. Rather, it's important to recognize the evident downsides of trauma, the
costs to the patient's life situation and the pain of psychic suffering,[85] particularly
early in treatment.

Yet posttraumatic growth is in some respects consonant with the IPT approach.
The results of the study just described support this. Later in treatment, if the patient is improving, learning new skills, and in fact taking appropriate control of a
not always fully controllable situation, it's worth pointing out how well the patient
is handling such a challenging situation. (This will invariably be a much better
outcome than the demoralized patient had been anticipating.) Many patients with
PTSD who improve in IPT (among other treatments) come to see themselves as
survivors, tougher and more sure of themselves for having come through a horrific
experience. Reinforcing positive patient adaptations has evident clinical benefit.

Most people will weather the extended crisis of Covid-19 without the need
for psychiatric intervention. A huge number, however, may need treatment.
We don't yet know what may be the optimal treatment approach(es) for many
Covid survivors; we need comparative clinical outcome studies to determine that.
I hope, however, that this book has made a convincing preliminary argument for
IPT as an appropriate approach.

ACKNOWLEDGMENTS

I must start by thanking the patients I have treated and whose cases I have supervised in the course of this painful pandemic. I thank Sarah Harrington for her editorial support and encouragement of this project at Oxford University Press. I thank my collaborative colleagues in the Military Family Wellness Center and the Anxiety Disorders Clinic at Columbia University/New York State Psychiatric Institute, who have been such a pleasure to work with before and during the pandemic, and especially Yuval Neria, PhD, Director of the Trauma and PTSD Program, who facilitated much of this research. Most of all, I thank my wife and infinitely patient colleague Barbara Milrod, MD, who supported my writing this book and contributed helpful insights to its final form.

John C. Markowitz, MD

REFERENCES

1. Centers for Disease Control and Prevention: *Anxiety and Depression: Household Pulse Survey.* https://www.cdc.gov/nchs/covid19/pulse/mental-health.htm
2. Markowitz JC, Milrod B, Heckman TG, Bergman M, Amsalem D, Zalman H, Ballas T, Neria Y: On remote: psychotherapy at a distance. *Am J Psychiatry* 2020;177. Epub ahead of print Sep 25.
3. Markowitz JC: *Interpersonal Psychotherapy for Posttraumatic Stress Disorder.* New York: Oxford University Press, 2016.
4. Kessler RC, Sonnega A, Bromet E, Hughes M, Nelson CB: Posttraumatic stress disorder in the National Comorbidity Survey. *Arch Gen Psychiatry* 1995;52:1048–1060.
5. Markowitz JC, Milrod B, Bleiberg KL, Marshall RD: Interpersonal factors in understanding and treating posttraumatic stress disorder. *J Psychiatr Practice* 2009;15:133–140.
6. Markowitz JC: Virtual treatment and social distancing. *Lancet Psychiatry* 2020;7:388–389.
7. Weissman MM, Markowitz JC, Klerman GL: *The Guide to Interpersonal Psychotherapy.* New York: Oxford University Press, 2018.
8. Cuijpers P, Geraedts AS, van Oppen P, Andersson G, Markowitz JC, van Straten A: Interpersonal psychotherapy of depression: a meta-analysis. *Am J Psychiatry* 2011;168:581–592.
9. Frank E, Kupfer DJ, Thase ME, Mallinger AG, Swartz HA, Fagiolini AM, Grochocinski V, Houck P, Scott J, Thompson W, Monk T: Two-year outcomes for interpersonal and social rhythm therapy in individuals with bipolar I disorder. *Arch Gen Psychiatry* 2005;62:996–1004.
10. Markowitz JC, Petkova E, Neria Y, Van Meter P, Zhao Y, Hembree E, Lovell K, Biyanova T, Marshall RD: Is exposure necessary? A randomized clinical trial of interpersonal psychotherapy for PTSD. *Am J Psychiatry* 2015;172;430–440.
11. Department of Veterans Affairs, Department of Defense. *VA/DoD Clinical Practice Guideline for the Management of Posttraumatic Stress Disorder and Acute Stress Disorder.* 2017. https://www.healthquality.va.gov/guidelines/MH/ptsd/VADoDPTSDCPGFinal012418.pdf
12. Markowitz JC, Friedman RA: NIMH's straight and neural path: the road to killing clinical psychiatric research. *Psychiatr Serv* 2020;71(11):1096–1097. Epub ahead of print Sep 23.

13. Milrod B, Keefe JR, Choo T-H, Arnon S, Such S, Lowell A, Neria Y, Markowitz JC: Separation anxiety in PTSD: a pilot prevalence and treatment study. *Depress Anxiety* 2020;37:386–395.

14. Markowitz JC, Lowell A, Milrod BL, Lopez-Yianilos A, Neria Y: Symptom-specific reflective function as a potential predictor of IPT outcome: a case report. *Am J Psychother* 2020;73(1):35–40. Epub ahead of print 6 Jan.

15. Frank E: *Treating Bipolar Disorder: A Clinician's Guide to Interpersonal and Social Rhythms Therapy.* New York: Guilford Press, 2007.

16. Brooks D: The first invasion of America. *New York Times* 2020 22 May. https://www.nytimes.com/2020/05/21/opinion/us-coronavirus-history.html?searchResultPosition=1

17. American Psychiatric Association: *Diagnostic and Statistical Manual of Mental Disorders*, Fifth Edition. Arlington, VA: American Psychiatric Association, 2013.

18. Williamson V, Murphy D, Greenberg N: Covid-19 and experiences of moral injury in front-line key workers. *Occup Med* 2020;70:317–319.

19. Ehlers CL, Frank E, Kupfer DJ: Social zeitgebers and biological rhythms. A unified approach to understanding the etiology of depression. *Arch Gen Psychiatry* 1988;45:948–952.

20. Newman A: What New York City sounds like every night at 7. *New York Times* 2010 10 Apr. https://www.nytimes.com/interactive/2020/04/10/nyregion/nyc-7pm-cheer-thank-you-coronavirus.html

21. Brewin CR, Andrews B, Valentine JD: Meta-analysis of risk factors for posttraumatic stress disorder in trauma-exposed adults. *J Consult Clin Psychol* 2000;68:748–766.

22. Ozer EJ, Best SR, Lipsey TL, Weiss DS: Predictors of posttraumatic stress disorder and symptoms in adults: a meta-analysis. *Psychol Bull* 2003;129:52–73.

23. National Academies of Sciences, Engineering, and Medicine: *Social Isolation and Loneliness in Older Adults: Opportunities for the Health Care System.* Washington, DC: National Academies Press, 2020. https://doi.org/10.17226/2566

24. Gao J, Zheng P, Jia Y, Chen H, May Y, Chen S, Wang Y, fu H, Dai J: Mental health problems and social media exposure during COVID-19 outbreak. *PLoS One* 2020;15(4):e0231924. doi:10.1371/journal.pone.0231924

25. Marino C, Gini G, Vieno A, Spada MM: The associations between problematic Facebook use, psychological distress and well-being among adolescents and young adults: a systematic review and meta-analysis. *J Affect Disord* 2018;226:274–281.

26. Shensa A, Escobar-Viera CG, Sidani JE, Bowman ND, Marshal MP, Primack BA: Problematic social media use and depressive symptoms among U.S. young adults: a nationally representative study. *Soc Sci Med* 2017;182:150–157.

27. Escobar-Viera CG, Shensa A, Bowman ND, Sidani JE, Knight J, James AE, Primack BA: Passive and active social media use and depressive symptoms among United States adults. *Cyberpsychol Behav Soc Netw* 2018;21:437–443.

28. Lee-Won R, Herzog L. Park S: Hooked on Facebook: the role of social anxiety and need for social assurance in problematic use of Facebook. *Cyberpsychol Behav Social Network* 2015;18. doi:10.1089/cyber.2015.0002

29. Shensa A, Sidani JE, Dew MA, Escobar-Viera CG, Primack BA: Social media use and depression and anxiety symptoms: a cluster analysis. *Am J Health Behav* 2018;42:116–128.

30. Primack BA, Shensa A, Sidani JE, Whaite EO, Lin LY, Rosen D, Colditz JB, Radovid A, Miller E: Social media use and perceived social isolation among young adults in the U.S. *Am J Prev Med* 2017;53:1–8.

31. Luxton DD, June JD, Fairall JM: Social media and suicide: a public health perspective. *Am J Public Health* 2012;102:S195–S200. doi:10.2105/AJPH.2011.300608

32. Amsalem D, Dixon L, Neria Y: The COVID-19 outbreak and mental health: current risks and recommended actions. *JAMA Psychiatry* 2020 24 Jun. doi:10.1001/jamapsychiatry.2020.1730. Online ahead of print.

33. Lowell A, Suarez-Jimenez B, Helpman L, Zhu X, Durosky A, Hilburn A, Schneier F, Fross R, Neria Y: 9/11-related PTSD among highly exposed populations: a systematic review 15 years after the attack. *Psychol Med* 2018;48:537–553.

34. Ferrando SJ, Klepacz L, Lynch S, Tavakkoli M, Dornbush R, Baharani R, Smolin Y, Bartell A: COVID-19 psychosis: a potential new neuropsychiatric condition triggered by novel coronavirus infection and the inflammatory response? *Psychosomatics* 2020;61:551–555.

35. Top ER doctor who treated virus patients dies by suicide. *New York Times* 2020 27 Apr. https://www.nytimes.com/2020/04/27/nyregion/new-york-city-doctor-suicide-coronavirus.html

36. Roose SP, Glick RA: *Anxiety as Symptom and Signal*. New York: Taylor & Francis, 2013.

37. Palacio CG, Krikorian A, Gomez-Romero MJ, Limonero JT: Resilience in caregivers: a systematic review. *Am J Hosp Palliat Care* 2020;28:3007–3013

38. Connor KM, Davidson JRT: Development of a new resilience scale: the Connor Davidson Resilience Scale. *Depress Anxiety* 2003;18:76–82.

39. Rosenberg AR: Cultivating deliberate resilience during the coronavirus disease 2019 pandemic. *JAMA Pediatrics* 2020; 1749:817–818.

40. Leach LS, Christensen H: A systematic review of telephone-based interventions for mental disorders. *J Telemed Telecare* 2006;12:122–129.

41. Heckman TG, Markowitz JC, Heckman BD, Woldu H, Anderson T, Lovejoy TI, Shen Y, Sutton M, Yarber W: A randomized clinical trial showing persisting reductions in depressive symptoms in HIV-infected rural adults following brief telephone-administered interpersonal psychotherapy. *Ann Behav Med* 2018;52:299–308.

42. Cuijpers P, Berking M, Andersson G, et al: A meta-analysis of cognitive-behavioural therapy for adult depression, alone and in combination with other treatments. *Can J Psychiatry* 2013;58:376–385.

43. Elkin I, Shea MT, Watkins JT, et al: National Institute of Mental Health treatment of depression collaborative research program: general effectiveness of treatments. *Arch Gen Psychiatry* 1989;46:971–982.

44. Pew Research Center: *Mobile Fact Sheet* 2019 12 Jun. http://www.pewinternet.org/fact-sheet/mobile/

45. Aslop T: *Percentage of U.S. Households that Have a Computer from 1984 to 2016.* 2020 12 May. https://www.statista.com/statistics/214641/household-adoption-rate-of-computer-in-the-us-since-1997/

46. Anderson M, Perrin A, Jiang J, Kumar M: *10% of Americans Don't Use the Internet: Who Are They?* Pew Research Center 2019 22 Apr. https://www.pewresearch.org/fact-tank/2019/04/22/some-americans-dont-use-the-internet-who-are-they/

47. https://www.nytimes.com/2020/04/09/opinion/sunday/coronavirus-inequality-america.html?action=click&module=RelatedLinks&pgtype=Article

48. The corona virus may have reminded Americans that they're all in it together. But it has also showed them how dangerously far apart they are. *New York Times* 2020 9 Apr. https://www.nytimes.com/2020/04/09/opinion/sunday/inequality-coronavirus.html?referringSource=articleShare

49. McClellan MJ, Florell D, Palmer J, et al: Clinician telehealth attitudes in a rural community mental health center setting. *J Rural Ment Health* 2020;44:62–73.

50. Lowell A, Lopez-Yianilos A, Ryba M, et al: A university-based mental health center for veterans and their families: challenges and opportunities. *Psychiatr Serv* 2019;70:159–162

51. Pickover A, Lowell A, Lazarov A, Lopez-Yianilos A, Sanchez-Lacay A, Ryba M, Arnon S, Neria Y, Markowitz JC: Interpersonal psychotherapy for veterans and family members: an open trial. *Psychiatr Serv* 2020 17 May.

52. Anderson T, McClintock A, McCarrick S, et al: Working alliance, interpersonal problems, and depressive symptoms in tele-interpersonal psychotherapy for HIV-infected rural persons: evidence for an indirect effects model. *J Clin Psychol* 2018;74:286–303.

53. Mulligan J, Haddock G, Hartley S, et al: An exploration of the therapeutic alliance within a telephone-based cognitive behaviour therapy for individuals with experience of psychosis. *Psychol Psychother* 2014;87:393–410.

54. Reese RJ, Conoley CW, Brossart DF: Effectiveness of telephone counseling: a field-based investigation. *J Counsel Psychol* 2002;49:233–242.

55. Simon M; Women and the hidden burden of the corona virus. *Changing America* 2020 19 May. https://thehill.com/changing-america/respect/equality/488509-the-hidden-burden-of-the-coronavirus-on-women

56. Morrison S. Zoom responds to its privacy (and porn) problems. *Vox* 2020 2 Apr. https://www.vox.com/recode/2020/3/31/21201019/zoom-coronavirus-privacy-hacks

57. Turgoose D, Ashwick R, Murphy D: Systematic review of lessons learned from delivering tele-therapy to veterans with post-traumatic stress disorder. *J Telemed Telecare* 2018;24:575–585.

58. Liu L, Thorp SR, Moreno L, Wells SY, Glassman LH, Busch AC, Zamora T, Rodgers CS, Allard CB, Agha Z: Videoconferencing psychotherapy for veterans with PTSD: results from a randomized controlled non-inferiority trial. *J Telemed Telecare* 2020;26:507–519

59. Dettore D, Pozza A, Andersson G: Efficacy of technology-delivered cognitive behavioural therapy for OCD vs. control conditions, and in comparison with therapist-administered CBT: meta-analysis of randomized clinical trials. *Cogn Behav Ther* 2015;44:190–211.

60. Reger MA, Stanley IH, Joiner TE: Suicide mortality and coronavirus disease 2019—a perfect storm? *JAMA Psychiatry* 2020 10 Apr. Online ahead of print. doi:10.1001/jamapsychiatry.2020.1060

61. O'Leary A, Jalloh MF, Neria Y: Fear and culture: contextualising mental health impact of the 2014–2016 Ebola epidemic in West Africa. *BMJ Glob Health* 2018;3:e000924. doi:10.1136/ bmjgh-2018-000924

62. Neria Y, DiGrande L, Adams BG: Posttraumatic stress disorder following the September 11, 2001 terrorist attacks: a review of the literature among highly exposed populations. *Am Psychologist* 2011;66:429–446.

63. Busch F, Milrod B, Chen C, Singer M: *Trauma-Focused Psychodynamic Psychotherapy: Bringing Evidence-Based Psychodynamic Treatment to Patients with PTSD*. New York: Oxford University Press, in press.

64. Hilty DM, Cobb HC, Neufeld JD, et al: Telepsychiatry reduces geographic physician disparity in rural settings, but is it financially feasible because of reimbursement? *Psychiatr Clin North Am* 2008:31:85–94.

65. Kocsis JH, Leon AC, Markowitz JC, Manber R, Arnow B, Klein DN, Thase ME: Patient preference as a moderator of outcome for chronic depression treated with nefazodone, cognitive behavioral analysis system of psychotherapy, or their combination. *J Clin Psychiatry* 2009;70:354–361.

66. Markowitz JC, Meehan KB, Petkova E, Zhao Y, Van Meter PE, Neria Y, Pessin H, Nazia Y: Treatment preferences of psychotherapy patients with chronic PTSD. *J Clin Psychiatry* 2016;77:363–370.

67. Wickland E; Feds OK interstate licensing, paving way for telehealth expansion. *mHealth Intelligence* 2020 19 Mar. https://mhealthintelligence.com/news/feds-ok-interstate-licensing-paving-way-for-telehealth-expansion

68. Markowitz JC, Kocsis JH, Fishman B, Spielman LA, Jacobsberg LB, Frances AJ, Klerman GL, Perry SW: Treatment of depressive symptoms in human immunodeficiency virus-positive patients. *Arch Gen Psychiatry* 1998;55:452–457.

69. Klerman GL, Weissman MM, Rounsaville BJ, Chevron ES: *Interpersonal Psychotherapy for Depression*. New York: Basic Books, 1984.

70. Lipsitz J, Markowitz JC: Interpersonal theory, in *American Psychological Association Handbook of Clinical Psychology*. Edited by Norcross JC, VanderBos GR, Freedheim DK. Washington, DC: American Psychological Association, 2016, 183–212.

71. Cuijpers P, Donker T, Weissman MM, Ravitz P, Cristea IA: Interpersonal psychotherapy for mental health problems: a comprehensive meta-analysis. *Am J Psychiatry* 2016;173:680–687.

72. Markowitz JC, Lipsitz J, Milrod BL: A critical review of outcome research on interpersonal psychotherapy for anxiety disorders. *Depress Anxiety* 2014; 31:316–325.

73. Markowitz JC, Kocsis JH, Bleiberg KL, Christos PJ, Sacks MH: A comparative trial of psychotherapy and pharmacotherapy for "pure" dysthymic patients. *J Affect Disord* 2005;89:167–175.

74. Weissman MM, Klerman GL, Prusoff BA, Sholomskas D, Padian N: Depressed outpatients: results one year after treatment with drugs and/or interpersonal psychotherapy. *Arch Gen Psychiatry* 1981;38:51–55.

75. Frank E, Kupfer DJ, Perel JM, Cornes C, Jarrett DB, Mallinger AG, Thase ME, McEachran AB, Grochocinski VJ: Three-year outcomes for maintenance therapies in recurrent depression. *Arch Gen Psychiatry* 1990;47:1093–1099.

76. Frank E, Kupfer DJ, Buysse DJ, Swartz HA, Pilkonis PA, Houck PR, Rucci P, Novick DM, Grochocinski VJ, Stapf DM: Randomized trial of weekly, twice-monthly, and monthly interpersonal psychotherapy as maintenance treatment for women with recurrent depression. *Am J Psychiatry* 2007;164:761–767.

77. Parsons T: Illness and the role of the physician: a sociological perspective. *Am J Orthopsychiatry* 1951;21:452–460.

78. Hamilton M: A rating scale for depression. *J Neurol Neurosurg Psychiatry* 1960;25:56–62.

79. Beck AT, Steer RA, Brown GK: *Manual for the Beck Depression Inventory-II*. San Antonio, TX: Psychological Corporation, 1996.

80. Weathers FW, Blake DD, Schnurr PP, Kaloupek DG, Marx BP, Keane TM: *The Clinician-Administered PTSD Scale for DSM-5 (CAPS-5)*. 2013. www.ptsd.va.gov.

81. Weathers FW, Litz BT, Keane TM, Palmieri PA, Marx BP, Schnurr PP: *The PTSD Checklist for DSM-5 (PCL-5)*. 2013. www.ptsd.va.gov

82. Hamilton M: The assessment of anxiety states by rating. *Br J Med Psychol* 1959;32:50–55.

83. Markowitz JC, Swartz HA: Case formulation in interpersonal psychotherapy of depression, in *Handbook of Psychotherapy Case Formulation*, Second Edition. Edited by Eells TD. New York: Guilford Press, 2007, 221–250.

84. Krupnick JL, Sotsky SM, Simmens S, Moyer J, Elkin I, Watkins J, Pilkonis PA: The role of the therapeutic alliance in psychotherapy and pharmacotherapy outcome: findings in the National Institute of Mental Health Treatment of Depression Collaborative Research Program. *J Consult Clin Psychol* 1996;64:532–539.

85. Markowitz JC, Milrod B: The importance of responding to negative affect in psychotherapies. *Am J Psychiatry* 2011;168:124–128.

86. Markowitz JC, Milrod BL: Personal view: what to do when a psychotherapy fails. *Lancet Psychiatry* 2015;2:186–190.

87. Reynolds CF, Frank E, Perel JM, Imber SD, Cornes C, Miller MD, Mazumdar S, Houck PR, Dew MA, Stack JA, Pollock BG, Kupfer DJ: Nortriptyline and interpersonal psychotherapy as maintenance therapies for recurrent major depression: a randomized controlled trial in patients older than 59 years. *JAMA* 1999;28:39–45.

88. Irish LA, Kline CE, Gunn HE, Buysse DJ, Hall MH: The role of sleep hygiene in promoting public health: a review of empirical evidence. *Sleep Med Rev* 2015;22:23–36.

89. American Sleep Association. *Sleep Hygiene Tips*. https://www.sleepassociation.org/about-sleep/sleep-hygiene-tips/

90. Kvan S, Kleppe CL, Nordhus IH, Hovland A: Exercise as a treatment for depression: a meta-analysis. *J Affect Disord* 2016;202:67–86.

91. Swartz HA, Rucci P, Thase ME, Wallace M, Carretta E, Celedonia KL, Frank E: Psychotherapy alone and combined with medication as treatments for bipolar II depression: a randomized controlled trial. *J Clin Psychiatry* 2018;79:(2):16m11027. doi:10.4088/JCP.16m11027

92. Frank E, Hlastala S, Ritenour A, Houck P, Tu XM, Monk TH, Mallinger AG, Kupfer DJ: Inducing lifestyle regularity in recovering bipolar disorder patients: results from the maintenance therapies in bipolar disorder protocol. *Biol Psychiatry* 1997;41:1165–1173.

93. Goldbaum C; Can 8 million daily users be lured back to N.Y. mass transit? *New York Times* 2020 8 Jun. https://www.nytimes.com/2020/06/01/nyregion/coronavirus-commute-nyc-subway-cars.html?searchResultPosition=2

94. Cuijpers P, Noma H, Karyotaki E, Vinkers CH, Cipriani A, Furukawa TA: A network meta-analysis of the effects of psychotherapies, pharmacotherapies and their combination in the treatment of adult depression. *World Psychiatry* 2020;19:92–107.

95. Markowitz JC, Milrod B, Luytens P, Holmqvist R: Mentalizing in interpersonal psychotherapy. *Am J Psychother* 2019;72:95–100.

96. Markowitz JC: Psychotherapy and eclecticism. *Psychiatr Serv* 2005;56:612.

97. Klass ET, Milrod BL, Leon AC, Kay S, Schwalberg M, Markowitz JC: Does interpersonal loss preceding panic disorder onset moderate response to psychotherapy? *J Clin Psychiatry* 2009;70:406–411.

98. Prochaska JO, DiClemente CC: Stages and processes of self change in smoking: toward an integrative model of change. *J Consult Clin Psychol* 1983;5:390–395.

99. Frank J: Therapeutic factors in psychotherapy. *Am J Psychother* 1971; 25:350–361.

100. Holmes TH, Rahe RH: The Social Readjustment Rating Scale. *J Psychosom Res* 1967;11:213–218.

101. Freud S: Mourning and melancholia, in *The Standard Edition of the Complete Psychological Works of Sigmund Freud, Volume XIV (1914–1916): On the History of the Psycho-Analytic Movement, Papers on Metapsychology and Other Works*. 1917, 237–258. Edited (and translated) by Strachey J. London: Hogarth Press.

102. Markowitz JC: *Interpersonal Psychotherapy for Dysthymic Disorder*. Washington DC: American Psychiatric Press, 1998.

103. Bonanno GA, Galea S, Bucciarelli A, Vlahov D: What predicts psychological resilience after disaster? The role of demographics, resources, and life stress. *J Consult Clin Psychol* 2007;75:671–682

104. Marshall RD, Olfson M, Hellman F, Blanco C, Guardino M, Stuening E: Comorbidity, impairment, and suicidality in subthreshold PTSD. *Am J Psychiatry* 2001;158;1467–1473.

105. Wang PS, Berglund P, Olfson M, Pincus HA, Wells KB, Kessler RC: Failure and delay in initial treatment contact after first onset of mental disorders in the National Comorbidity Survey Replication. *Arch Gen Psychiatry* 2005;62:603–613.

106. Bleiberg KL, Markowitz JC: Interpersonal psychotherapy for posttraumatic stress disorder. *Am J Psychiatry* 2005;162:181–183.

107. *Using the PTSD Checklist for DCM-5 (PCL-5)*. Washington, DC: National Center for PTSD. https://www.ptsd.va.gov/professional/assessment/documents/using-PCL5.pdf

108. Steenkamp MM, Litz BT, Marmar CR: First-line psychotherapies for military-related PTSD. *JAMA* 2020;323:656–657.

109. Foa EB, Rothbaum BO: *Treating the Trauma of Rape: Cognitive-Behavioral Therapy for PTSD*. New York, Guilford Press, 1998.

110. Jacobsen E: *Progressive Relaxation*. Chicago: University of Chicago Press, 1938.

111. Markowitz JC, Neria Y, Lovell K, Van Meter PE, Petkova E: History of sexual trauma moderates psychotherapy outcome for posttraumatic stress disorder. *Depress Anxiety* 2017;34:692–700.

112. Markowitz JC, Choo T, Neria Y: Stability of improvement after psychotherapy of posttraumatic stress disorder. *Can J Psychiatry/La Revue canadienne de psychiatrie* 2018;63:37–43.

113. Krupnick JL, Green BL, Stockton P, Miranda J, Krause E, Mete M: Group interpersonal psychotherapy for low-income women with posttraumatic stress disorder. *Psychother Res* 2008; 18:497–507.

114. Campanini RF, Schoedl AF, Pupo MC, Costa AC, Krupnick JL, Mello MF: Efficacy of interpersonal therapy-group format adapted to post-traumatic stress disorder: an open-label add-on trial. *Depress Anxiety* 2010;27:72–77.

115. Lanius RA, Vermetten E, Lowenstein RJ, Brand B, Schmahl C, Bremner JD, Spiegel D: Emotion modulation in PTSD: clinical and neurobiological evidence for a dissociative subtype. *Am J Psychiatry* 2010;167:640–647.

116. Resick PA, Uhlmansiek MO, Clum GA, Galovski, TE, Scher CD, Yinong Y-X: A randomized clinical trial to dismantle components of cognitive processing therapy for posttraumatic stress disorder in female victims of interpersonal violence. *J Clin Consult Psychol* 2008;76:243–258.

117. Shapiro F: *Eye Movement Desensitization and Reprocessing (EMDR) Therapy*, Third Edition. New York: Guilford Press, 2017.

118. Brady K, Pearlstein T, Asnis GM, Baker D, Rothbaum B, Sikes CR, Farfel GM: Efficacy and safety of sertraline treatment of posttraumatic stress disorder: a randomized controlled trial. *JAMA* 2000;283:1837–1844.

119. Marshall RD, Beebe KL, Oldham M, Zaninelli R: Efficacy and safety of paroxetine treatment for chronic PTSD: a fixed-dose, placebo-controlled study. *Am J Psychiatry* 2001;158:1982–1988.

120. Raskind MA, Peskind ER, Chow B, Harris C, Davis-Karim A, Holmes HA, Hart KL, McFall M, Mellman TA, Reist C, Romesser J, Rosenheck R, Shih M-C, Stein MB, Swift R, Gleason T, Lu Y, Huang GD: Trial of prazosin for post-traumatic stress disorder in military veterans. *N Engl J Med* 2018;378:507–517.

121. Schneier FR, Neria Y, Pavlicova M, Hembree E, Suh EJ, Amsel L, Marshall RD: Combined prolonged exposure therapy and paroxetine for PTSD related to the World Trade Center attack: a randomized controlled trial. *Am J Psychiatry* 2012;169:80–88.

122. Litz BT, Stein N, Delaney E, Lebowitz L, Nash WP, Silva C, Maguen S: Moral injury and moral repair in war veterans: a preliminary model and intervention strategy. *Clin Psychol Rev* 2009;29:695–706.

123. Cividanes GC, Mello AF, Mello MF: Revictimization as a high-risk factor for development of posttraumatic stress disorder: a systematic review of the literature. *Braz J Psychiatry* 2019;41:82–89.

124. Busch FN, Milrod BL, Singer MB, Aronson AC: *Manual of Panic-Focused Psychodynamic Psychotherapy—eXtended range*. New York: Routledge/Taylor & Francis, 2012.

125. Karam AM, Fitzsimmons-Craft EE, Tanofsky-Kraff M, Wilfley DE: Interpersonal psychotherapy and the treatment of eating disorders. *Psychiatr Clin North Am* 2019;42:205–218.

126. Working Group on Eating Disorders. *Practice Guideline for the Treatment of Patients With Eating Disorders*, Third Edition. Washington, DC: American Psychiatric Association, 2010. https://psychiatryonline.org/pb/assets/raw/sitewide/practice_guidelines/guidelines/eatingdisorders.pdf

127. Beck AT, Brown G, Epstein N, Steer RA: An inventory for measuring clinical anxiety: psychometric properties. *J Consult Clin Psychol* 1988;56:893–897.

128. Ruiz NG, Horowitz JM, Tamir C: *Many Black and Asian Americans Say They Have Experienced Discrimination Amid the COVID-19 Outbreak*. Pew Research Center 2010 10 Jul. https://www.pewsocialtrends.org/2020/07/01/many-black-and-asian-americans-say-they-have-experienced-discrimination-amid-the-covid-19-outbreak/

129. Judd LL, Akiskal HS, Maser JD, Zeller PJ, Endicott J, Coryell W, Paulus MP, Kunovac JL, Leon AC, Mueller TI, Rice JA, Keller MB: A prospective 12–year study of subsyndromal and syndromal depressive symptoms in unipolar major depressive disorders. *Arch Gen Psychiatry* 1998;55:694–700.

130. Judd LL, Akiskal HS: Delineating the longitudinal structure of depressive illness: beyond clinical subtypes and duration thresholds. *Pharmacopsychiatry* 2000;1:3–7.

131. Cyranowski JM, Frank E, Winter E, Rucci P, Novick D, Pilkonis P, Fagiolini A, Swartz HA, Houck P, Kupfer DJ: Personality pathology and outcome in recurrently depressed women over two years of maintenance interpersonal psychotherapy. *Psychol Med* 2004;34:659–669.

132. *The Compact Oxford English Dictionary*, Second Edition. Oxford: Clarendon Press, 1991, 1568/714.

133. Rusch HL, Shvil E, Szanton SL, Neria Y, Gill JM: Determinants of psychological resistance and recovery among women exposed to assaultive trauma. *Brain Behav* 2015 Apr;5(4):e00322. doi:10.1002/brb3.322

134. Southwick SM, Bonnano GA, Masten AS, Panter-Brick C, Yehuda R: Resilience definitions, theory, and challenges: interdisciplinary perspectives. *Eur J Psychotraumatol* 2014;5:10.3402/ejpt.v5.25338. doi:10.3402/ejpt.v5.25338

135. Bowlby JL: *Attachment and Loss*. London: Hogarth, 1969.

136. Bowlby J: Attachment and loss: retrospect and prospect. *Am J Orthopsychiatry* 1982;52:664–678.

137. Brewin CR, Andrews B, Valentine JD: Meta-analysis of risk factors for posttraumatic stress disorder in trauma-exposed adults. *J Consult Clin Psychol* 2000;68:748–766.

138. Ozer EJ, Best SR, Lipsey TL, Weiss DS: Predictors of posttraumatic stress disorder and symptoms in adults: a meta-analysis. *Psychol Bull* 2003;129:52–73.

139. Wilks CR, Morland LA, Dillon KH, Mackintosh MA, Blakey SM, Wagner HR; VA Mid-Atlantic MIRECC Workgroup, Elbogen EB: Anger, social support, and suicide risk in US military veterans. *J Psychiatric Res* 2019;109:139–144.

140. Cyranowski, JM, Shear MK, Rucci P, Fagiolini A, Frank E, Grochocinski VJ, Kupfer DJ, Banti S, Armani A, Cassano G: Adult separation anxiety: psychometric properties of a new structured clinical interview. *J Psychiatr Res* 2002;36:77–86.

141. Rudden MG, Milrod B, Meehan KB, Falkenstrom F: Symptom-specific reflective functioning: incorporating psychoanalytic measures into clinical trials. *J Am Psychoanal Assoc* 2009;57:1473–1478.

142. Rudden M, Milrod B, Target M, Ackerman S, Graf E: Reflective functioning in panic disorder patients: a pilot study. *J Am Psychoanal Assn* 2006;54:1339–1343.

143. Silove D, Ionso J, Bromet E, Gruber M, Sampson N, Scott K, Andrade L, Benjet C, Caldas de Almeida JM, De Girolamo G, de Jonge P, Demyttenaere K, Fiestas F, Florescu S, Gureje O, He Y, Karam E, Lepine JP, Murphy S, Villa-Posada J, Zarkov Z, Kessler RC: Pediatric-onset and adult-onset separation anxiety disorder across countries in the World Mental Health Survey. *Am J Psychiatry* 2015;172;647–656.

144. Bernstein M, Pfefferbaum B: Posttraumatic growth as a response to natural disasters in children and adolescents. *Curr Psychiatry Rep* 2018;20(5):37. doi:10.1007/s11920-018-0900-4

For the benefit of digital users, indexed terms that span two pages (e.g., 52–53) may, on occasion, appear on only one of those pages.

Tables, figures and boxes are indicated by *t*, *f* and *b* following the page number